"Dr. Maita has spent decades understanding the human body. This is a great operating manual for everyone who wants well-informed, sensible advice about how to live, not just to age. Unlike all the confusing advice on-line, Dr. Maita has edited this book down to the basics you must know, stripped of all the fads."

~ Ronna Lichtenberg,
CEO, Videotrope

"This book is a must-read. Dr. Maita helps you tap into the inspiration and motivation to get you started and then gives clear and compelling reasons as to the what, why, and how to go about a comprehensive program to live a long healthy life. She's great and her book is great. Buy it and share it with everyone you care about."

~ Jim Donovan,
author, "52 Ways to a Happier Life"

"Dr. Lorraine Maita's new book, *"Vibrance for Life: How to Live Younger and Healthier"*, contains a wealth of knowledge in an easy-to-read format. In today's world, age 60 is the beginning of middle age. Dr. Maita's literary work gives the reader a bird's-eye view of ways to help one live to be a healthy 100 years. It is a must read for people of any age. "

~ Pamela W. Smith, M.D., MPH
*Co-Director, Masters Program in Medical Sciences
with a concentration in Metabolic and Nutritional Medicine,
University of South Florida College of Medicine*

"If you are looking for a book that can show you the way to create more good health and well-being in your life, I recommend this one. In *Vibrance for Life*, author and doctor Lorraine Maita effectively shares what it takes to have more energy, a slimmer body, and, most of all, an undeniable vibrancy others will be sure to notice! I particularly like the way the author asks questions that get at the very core about why a change wants to be made. It's also chock-full of straightforward information about good health habits and the way the body works. Maita has written an excellent book for people who care about their health and want to make some changes for the better!"

~ Donna Kozik,
Founder, MyBigBusinessCard.com

"The healthcare reform debate has completely missed the point: Seventy-five percent of healthcare spending in the U.S. goes toward treating preventable diseases. Notably, the declines that come with aging fall within this category as well. *Vibrance for Life* is a timely and unique book that highlights the importance of prevention as the only true healthcare reform – with sensible guidance for us to avoid the major causes of premature death, including diabetes, high blood pressure, and cardiovascular disease. And with nearly 12,000 Americans turning age 50 every day, this book couldn't come at a better time.

Vibrance for Life addresses the "practical stuff," the nuts and bolts efforts of which people need to be mindful. Dr. Maita offers a no-nonsense approach to place us on the road to good health and a better quality of life. This book is practical and is a must-read for anyone aspiring to vibrant health at any age."

~ Gregory Petersburg, DO
Founder and Author,
Living Younger Preventive-Aging Medicine & Business System

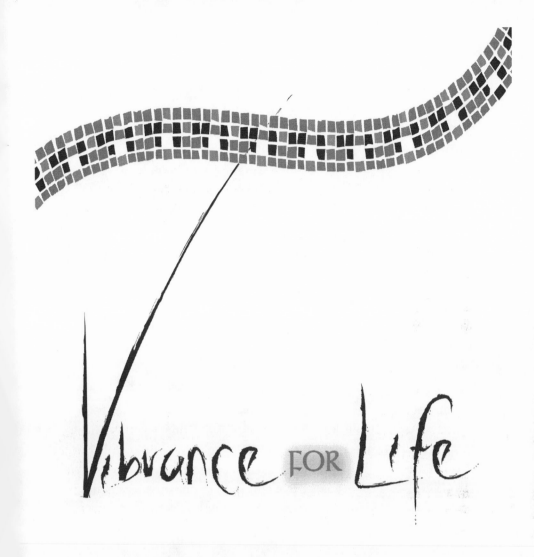

Vibrance for Life

How to Live Younger and Healthier

Lorraine Maita, MD

Editor: Jodi Brandon
Cover designer: Jodi Topitz
Typesetter: Susan Veach

Vibrance for Life
51 JFK Parkway, First Floor West
Short Hills, NJ 07078
info@howtoliveyounger.com
www.howtoliveyounger.com
www.vibranceforlife.com
ISBN# 978-0-9833148-0-6

Limits of Liability and Disclaimer of Warranty
The author and publisher shall not be liable for your misuse of this material. This book is strictly for informational and educational purposes.

Warning – Disclaimer
The purpose of this book is to educate and entertain. The author and/or publisher does not guarantee that anyone following these techniques, suggestions, tips, ideas, or strategies will become successful. The author and/or publisher shall have neither liability nor responsibility to anyone with respect to any loss or damage caused, or alleged to be caused, directly or indirectly by the information contained in this book. Unless otherwise noted, tables were created by the author after consulting with many OTC multivitamins, the RDA, and studies, as well as nutraceutical-grade multivitamins and books listed in the References.

The publisher and author are not responsible for any adverse effects or consequences resulting from the use of any of the suggestions, preparations, or procedures discussed in this book. The information and advice contained in this book are based upon the research and the personal and professional experience of the author. They are not intended as a substitute for consulting with a healthcare professional. All matters pertaining to your physical health should be supervised by a healthcare professional. It is a sign of wisdom, not cowardice, to seek a second or third opinion.

Dedication

This book is dedicated to my patients, mentors, and mother, who taught me a great deal and made me a better doctor. Without them, none of this would be possible, and I am grateful for their support.

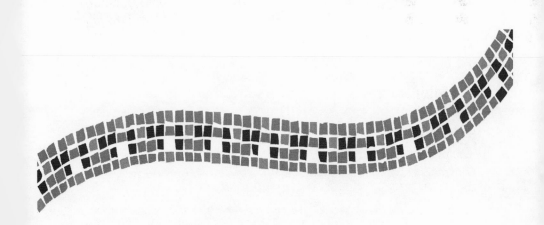

Acknowledgments

I would like to thank my my editor, Jodi Brandon, for her insights, dedication, and attention to detail and Jodi Topitz, my cover designer, for bringing an eye-catching life and vibrance to the cover.

I would also like to thank Pam Smith, MD, and my colleagues at the American Academy of Anti Aging and Regenerative Medicine, and Gregory Petersburg, DO, founder of the Living Younger program, for their support, knowledge, and expertise, and for making me a believer in the power of anti-aging medicine.

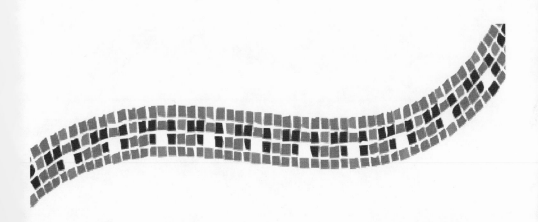

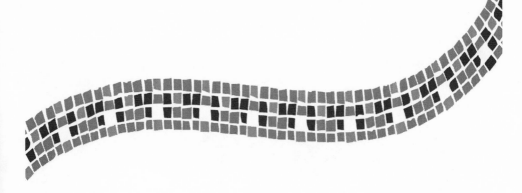

Contents

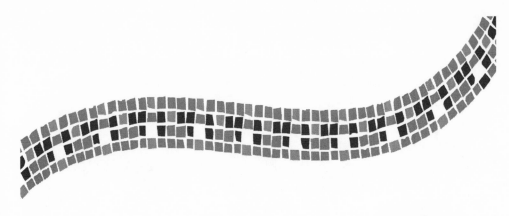

Preface

This book answers some of the questions that my patients ask most frequently. They become motivated when they know why they are doing something, since preventive medicine can sometimes take time before a difference is noticeable. The differences can be subtle and become apparent when comparing the initial complaints with present complaints.

Many books go into great depths on only one aspect of health. I could write a book about every chapter. However, harnessing the synergistic power of a comprehensive approach incorporating diet, exercise, supplements and hormones, and stress management has far greater effects, which is why I prefer to give you some simple steps to take where you will get the greatest impact. This is meant to be a quick and easy guide to get started. It's the CliffsNotes version. What I hope to achieve is to simplify complex metabolic processes and empower readers to get motivated to change. You can improve wherever you are at any age, and doing so does not require a lot of time, cost, or equipment. Sometimes a small change can make a big difference.

While there is no substitute for a detailed, customized approach using innovative genetic and metabolic tests to tailor treatment to an individual's unique metabolism, these simple measures can dramatically change your life and your health.

It is my greatest hope to help you achieve your health goals, live a vibrant, full life, and experience all of life's joys.

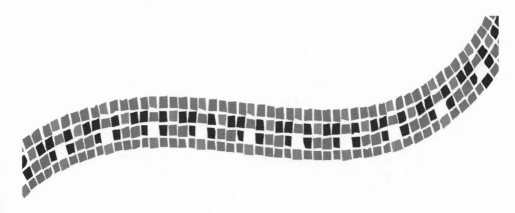

Introduction

Did you wake up one day, stiff, sore, tired, and forgetful, and wonder what happened to you? Or perhaps, the figure you look at in the mirror is fuller and rounder in certain spots, your skin has lost that youthful glow, and there is something not right. Your libido or energy may be low, or you may have a vague, listless feeling that you have lost something. *Where did I put those keys? What was so and so's name — you know, from where you used to work? What happened to my memory? Could it be Alzheimer's? And why don't I have the strength to lift those boxes anymore? There must be something wrong.*

You go to the doctor and have some tests run, and you are told that you are just getting old! *No, not those words, not me! I don't want to be old, lose my mobility, my memory, or my vision or other senses.* You go through all of the stages: anger, denial, bargaining — yet you feel that somewhere somehow there must be a better way. The bad news is that we are all aging from the moment we are born, and nothing short of death will stop that process.

Take a deep breath. The good news is that you can modulate the process. Aging doesn't have to be a rapid nosedive into a wheelchair and having a hearing aid, dentures, and poor sight. We are living much longer than previous generations, and are determined to make those years count and have the quality of life be a life worth living. We not only want to survive, we want to thrive.

There is so much to think about, and there are so many choices. The air is polluted and we can be prone to allergies. Our food and water are contaminated. Snake oil salesmen play to our fears, promising quick fixes and the fountain of youth or a magic bullet. There is a plethora of supplements and health aids, and it is difficult to separate the wheat from the chaff. It can seem so overwhelming.

Even as a medical professional who has dedicated my career to health, healing, and preventive medicine, the information overload of products, tests, medications, and programs is daunting. Sorting through to find what is scientifically valid and appropriate for someone can be difficult.

I worked in an emergency room and in hospitals in New York City, and I thought I saw it all. People came back over and over again with the same ailments. It was like the movie *Groundhog Day*. Even though I worked hard to treat and stabilize people, they would return again and again. I sometimes saw people suffer or die prematurely from something that could have been prevented, and I agonized over what I could do to make a difference.

A turning point for me was seeing a man with most of his fingers cut off and all of his toes cut off still smoking a cigarette. This was the very thing that caused the loss of his digits. It was sad and sobering that, even with the best medical care, we couldn't get through to him. I vowed to work hard to educate people, and motivate and inspire them to prevent illness — or to at least catch it early when it was treatable and didn't do any permanent damage.

So I studied and tried to apply the knowledge, and I learned that not everyone responded to the "best" treatment or the standard of care. I quickly learned we are all unique and looked for signs to unlock the secret code to how to prevent or treat chronic disease.

Anti-aging medicine is giving us more answers now. Each person metabolizes the same things differently based on genetics, lifestyle, environment, and hormonal, nutritional, and attitudinal status. The aging process is the same for everyone; it's how we respond to the process and how we determine what part of us is most likely to break down that hold the key.

This field of medicine is so exciting, because we are beginning to unlock the codes to how we age and how to slow the process. I get so excited when I see people turn their lives around every day and tell me that they feel great again. They have renewed energy and strength, they have sharper mental focus and improved memory, their weight comes off, their skin glows, and they feel great.

This can be you. With motivation and dedication, you *can* live younger. I will guide you through some of the basics you can do on your own. This advice is what I give to my patients. I hope to inspire you to seek medical guidance, adopt any or all of these practices to slow the aging process, and maintain the energy and vitality of youth so you can live your dream life, personally and professionally.

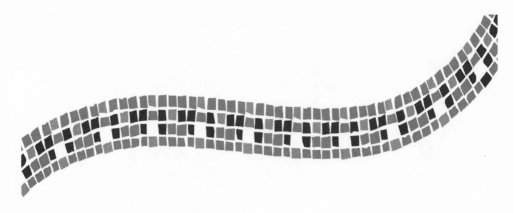

Chapter 1
Get Motivated

What's Motivating You?

What made you buy this book? Do you want to be inspired to have vibrant health no matter what your age is? Are you looking for simple ways in which you can improve your health and lead a more fulfilling life with energy, clarity, and self-confidence?

Congratulate yourself for taking that first step. I'll share with you the secrets and strategies that I use to work with my patients so you, too, can live younger and healthier. Developing the mindset, understanding your motivations, setting clear goals, and establishing a plan are keys to success, along with monitoring and tracking your progress. While it's best to have a professional who can guide you, hold you accountable, monitor your progress, and help you get past obstacles, I have kept this simple enough for you to follow on your own so you can benefit from improvements in your overall health. While this is not meant to diagnose or treat any underlying disease, these lifestyle modifications have shown proven benefits in the medical literature.

Can You Relate?

My knees hurt and I have fat around my midline, I am on blood pressure and cholesterol medication, my blood sugar is creeping up, and I don't want to die of a heart attack like my father.

My mother died of breast cancer and Alzheimer's runs in the family. I don't want that to be me.

I feel tired all of the time, I have no sex drive, and I am afraid my wife will leave me or I will lose my job.

The hot flashes are interfering with my sleep. I am tired and irritable, and can't have sex because I am so dry.

People come to me for many reasons. Some are sick and tired of being sick and tired. Others are on medications that have unpleasant side effects or they no longer want to be dependent on medication. Others are well and want to stay well because their parents or siblings suffered from diabetes, heart attack, stroke, cancer, or other illness. Some are in pain, either physical or emotional. The reasons you picked up this book or go to a doctor to seek help and guidance are varied, and it's these reasons that will keep you on your path. Writing them down and committing to them is important. Here's why.

I take notes and during every visit I ask patients what has changed. Here is a typical scenario:

What's different?

Really nothing. I am not feeling any better.

How is your sleep?

It's good. I sleep through the night.

Do you remember telling me that you would keep waking up and were not able to go back to sleep?

Oh yeah! Now I remember!

How is your energy level?

I am still tired.

Are you as tired as you had been, and do you still fall asleep at your desk in the afternoon?

Now that you mention it, no, I am not as tired. I am able to do more now. I don't get so exhausted that I pass out at my desk.

You get the picture. The changes are small, gradual, and not readily noticeable because *the ultimate* goal and vision have not yet been met. The subtle changes were not recognized as progress. Metabolic medicine is slower and less dramatic than taking a pharmaceutical drug. You may not notice the effects because they are so gradual. I often get phone calls from people saying they have been taking the supplements I recommended and don't feel better. When I ask how long they have been taking them and they say a few days, I smile inside. We are a culture of *now* — expecting fast results, a magic pill, and a quick fix.

The analogy I use is that of renovating a house, or a vintage or high-performance car. You have to go slowly, brick by brick, or the structure will collapse. It takes longer to renovate a house carefully than it takes to build one from scratch. Removing and replacing worn or damaged structures (cells and tissues) has to be done carefully with proper timing and order. The quality of the materials we use (food and supplements) is what will make the structure last and withstand stressors. An aging body is like owning a vintage car. A vintage car is exotic and beautiful, and it requires more maintenance. A high-performance car requires the proper fuel and maintenance to perform at its optimum with power and speed. You wouldn't dare put substandard oil or gas in such a classic. It's a labor of love to care for a house, or a vintage car, so love yourself and care for yourself in that way that you would a precious classic!

The point is that caring for something or someone we love comes from the heart, and the very act itself can be rewarding. Also, every bit of progress that you can monitor and track will keep you motivated. It's easy to forget how far you have come. The progress isn't always dramatic; it can be subtle and small, but nevertheless, if you are moving forward, you can gather momentum.

The Pleasure-Pain Principle

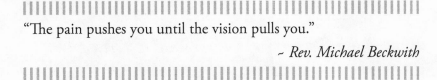

"The pain pushes you until the vision pulls you."

- Rev. Michael Beckwith

Your challenge is to create a clear vision of what your dream of success and health looks like that is so compelling that it gives you the energy and motivation to push through obstacles. You may have setbacks, and when the going gets rough you start telling yourself you weren't feeling that bad and that you really don't mind taking so many medications because it is easy. You convince yourself that some of the things you are experiencing are not so bad. This type of rationalization will set you back into old habits that will derail you. To develop new habits takes some time and effort. You can make it hard, or you can make it easy. Resistance can make it hard. A sense of curiosity, play, and experimentation will not only make it easier, it can make it fun.

Getting Ready: Assess

Motivational Self-Assessment: Are You Ready to Leap?

Answer these questions. These will serve as the foundation for what is motivating you to change. When you come across an obstacle or setback, you can refer to these to recapture the motivation and inspiration that got you started. (These are listed in Appendix I with room to write your answers.)

Where am I now?

- What am I most afraid of?
- What is bothering me the most?
- If I changed one thing, what would make the most difference in my life?

Where do I want to go?

- What does it look and feel like to reach my goal?

Why do I want this?

- What is my ultimate goal?
- Do I want to start small or get to the bottom of all of my issues more quickly?
- What am I willing to do to reach my goals?

Getting Set: Plan

Create a Vision

What will it look and feel like when I improve or reach my goals? How will it impact the different areas of my life?

- Physical
- Emotional
- Financial
- Social
- Other

Conceive it and Create a Compelling Vision

A vision is something lofty and big, not bound by our limiting beliefs. Stretch, and have fun with this. You can get more specific and realistic later. All things large and small start with a conception of them — a vision or picture in your mind. That vision can be something as simple as what you want for dinner or as big as creating an empire. Big or small, it starts with a thought.

This is your life, your health, your mind, and your body, and you are the master of your destiny. What do you want to create? Some ways to conceive of your being able to do this are to read or listen to inspiring stories about ordinary people who did extraordinary things. Oprah has gained such popularity and power by inspiring people and letting them tell their stories. This makes it real and makes it seem possible. Do whatever it takes to begin creating your vision. Just picking up this book is a good first step. Perhaps stories and news article about cutting-edge science would give you some inspiration. Dream and create your vision of health and how it will impact your life.

Examples: Ready, Set Go!

A 48-year-old overweight woman who is getting hot flashes, doesn't sleep well, and no longer feels desirable is on medication for sleep and high cholesterol. She is slightly depressed and wants to feel like herself again, as well as regain her self-esteem. Her vision might look like this:

My vision for my life and health are:

- I see myself 30 pounds lighter in a beautiful, form-fitting dress. I am cool and calm yet energetic. I feel sexy and vibrant. My sleep is deep, and I control my cholesterol with healthy food that I really enjoy. My activities are stimulating, make me feel good and I lose weight. I feel great and enjoy my newfound health and lifestyle. It is easy and effortless. Now I have the confidence and clarity to start that coaching business I have always wanted to, and I can write about my success and share it with others.

Achieving this vision will impact my life in the following ways:

- Physical — energy, better sleep, no medication side effects, fit into clothes

- Emotional — improved self-esteem and confidence opens more opportunities in both my personal and professional life

- Financial — decreased risk of heart attack and other disease related to weight, less money for medication and doctor's visits to monitor it; I can start a business that is both personally and financially fulfilling

- Social — better relationship with husband and children because I am sleeping better and more refreshed; I feel better able to get out and network for my business

- Other — in going through this process I am learning more about myself

A 52-year-old male is balding, developing a paunch, and lacks motivation. He is losing his edge at work due to his memory not being as sharp and clear. Stress levels are high, and he finds it hard to keep up. He was recently diagnosed with high blood pressure, and the medications are dampening his sex drive. He now has borderline diabetes and his joints ache, so he is tentative about exercise. All of this is demoralizing and he doesn't know where to start.

My vision for my life and health are:

- I see myself fit, mentally sharp and clear, and as competitive and capable as ever. I am trim and fit as well as energetic with a satisfying sex life. As the pounds slip away, I find I no longer need medication and my health is fantastic. Fitness and health have become my lifestyle, and the more I do, the more I am capable of doing. I ask for and get a promotion and can get that Porsche I always wanted. I have an ample amount of money to send my kids to a good college, which will relieve a lot of my stress.

Achieving this vision will impact my life in the following ways:

- Physical — mental quickness and clarity, competitive edge, strong, fit, energetic

- Emotional — improved self-esteem and confidence, less stress, better sexual relations with my wife

- Financial — I'll ask for that promotion and get make more money

- Social — status, family cared for

- Other — I feel like myself again and now want to do some philanthropic work

Goal-Setting

A lofty vision can seem overwhelming and unattainable unless you chunk it down into small steps or goals. Each chapter of this book focuses on a different area, and you can decide on steps for each area. No vision will carry you unless you believe it and know it is possible. The stories, the explanations, and the guidance in this book are meant to make a believer out of you. The more faith and belief you have in something, the more you will invest in it.

SMART Goals

To assure success in reaching your goals they must be SMART:

- **S**pecific
- **M**easurable
- **A**ttainable
- **R**ealistic
- **T**ime-Bound

There are tracking tools in the appendices to help you develop your goals. Here are some examples:

Food Choices

I will cut down on sugar and fat in my diet, and eat more vegetables.

- Week 1: cut out 1 soda and substitute water, take ½ tsp. sugar in coffee instead of 1 tsp., add 1 extra vegetable to lunch and dinner
- Week 2: no soda, ¼ tsp. sugar in coffee, no white foods, 1 less serving of red meat this week

Exercise

I will start to get more aerobic activity first and later add weights.

- Week 1: park car far away and walk 15 minutes before I get to my desk
- Week 2: walk 30 minutes
- Week 3: start weight routine with 1 set for each muscle group

Go: Action!

Assess: What's Aging You?

Knowing what your most vulnerable areas are can help you focus on your weakest part. You are only as young as your "oldest" part, and that part may fail first. Think of your health as an iceberg beneath the surface: There is a lot you can't see. You wake up one morning and you lose your balance and fall. You can't open a jar or see the fine-print anymore. The TV has to be turned up louder. Getting up the stairs is harder and painful.

Even without equipment or a professional to measure, there are some things you can assess on your own, and others you will need to ask your doctor for.

Visit Your Doctor

Get a baseline of your measurements to assess your risk for cardiovascular disease, obesity, and weight-related illness as well as to track progress. Here are some important numbers:

- Height
- Weight
- Blood pressure
- Pulse
- Body mass index (BMI)*
- Body composition (percent fat)
- Waist size
- Hip size
- Waist-to-hip ratio

*NOTE: Body mass index (BMI) is a relationship between weight and height that is associated with body fat and health risk.

Basic blood tests are essential to determine if you have any underlying illness and can be early indicators of risk for developing illness. Some basic tests that assess your metabolic function are:

- Fasting blood sugar
- Metabolic panel or chem. screen
- Complete blood count (CBC)
- Lipids (cholesterol, LDL, HDL, and triglycerides)

Advanced tests for cardiovascular disease and metabolic syndrome are emerging as important in determining risk for disease and can guide treatment options:

- Lipoprotein particle analysis
- C-Reactive Protein
- Homocysteine
- Fasting insulin
- Hemoglobin A1c

Other age- or gender-specific tests that are early markers for cancer, osteoporosis, and hormone deficiencies or imbalances are:

- Prostate specific antigen (PSA)
- Pap smear
- Mammography
- DEXA bone scan
- Hormone levels

Refer to the appendices to determine your risk and record your findings.

Prioritize

Knowing your personal risk factors can help you prioritize. Your doctor or a metabolic anti-aging specialist can help you find the common thread and assist you in focusing on the areas that will have the greatest impact. However, just following some basic lifestyle principles can improve your health.

Put your plan of action on paper or in your computer. Now you are ready to begin.

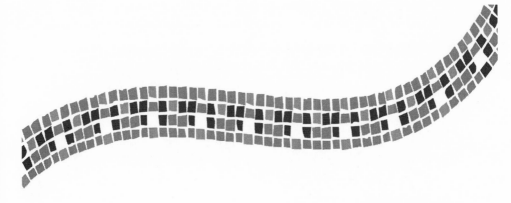

Chapter 2
Food as Medicine

Can You Relate?

Do you get gas, bloating, or fat around your midline? Do you have mental fog, minor aches, or nasal congestion?

> Nan, a 50-year-old woman, complained of fatigue, loss of clarity, and weight gain. She has a history of being allergic to several antibiotics but not to food. Her symptoms were vague, and she was found to be hypothyroid. However, once her thyroid hormone level was normalized, she still had vague feelings of not being herself, and she had a very hard time losing weight.
>
> Ernest, a 45-year-old man with high blood pressure and high cholesterol, had joint aches, mental fog, and listlessness. He complained of weight gain and felt that the medications he was on affected his libido. His testosterone levels were normalized, and he was demoralized by his lack of libido.

Food is such an integral part of life. It is a source of fuel, which is converted to energy for use by cells, tissues, and organs. Without it, you can't function. It is also used to celebrate, to comfort and console, to reward, to give us a physical or mental boost, or to fill time. Many social gatherings occur around a meal or food of some kind. Our society, due to the abundance of food, has moved away from "eat to live," to "live to eat." Food, however, can fuel or foul your system, depending on your choices, so let's look at food from a metabolic perspective. Food can accelerate or decelerate developing disease and/or the aging process.

Like anything in nature, we burn, brown, and rust, our hormones get out of balance, and our nervous systems decline. Metabolically, these processes are called glycation (browning), oxidation (rusting), and inflammation (burning). Neuro decline occurs when neurotransmitters, the chemical signals to our brain and nervous system, decline, are out of balance, or stop functioning. Hormones change as we age. Some hormones decline with age, while others get higher.

Inflammation is the redness and swelling that occurs with trauma or infection and any condition ending with "itis," like arthritis, gastritis, or gingivitis. Inflammation can be dramatic and give a clear signal, or it can be a low-grade, smoldering condition that is not easily detected. The inflammatory response increases as we age.

Medical literature links inflammation to many chronic diseases and may be a factor in accelerating the aging process. In 2004, *Time* magazine ran a cover story ("Inflammation: The Fires Within") on the research being done on inflammation as a causative factor in autoimmune disease, asthma, cancer, cardiovascular disease, diabetes, and Alzheimer's disease. Controlling inflammation may be the key to preventing and managing these and other diseases.

Glycation is like the browning of a sugar-coated ham: Sugar binds to proteins and "glycates" them. It's great to eat, but not if the process occurs in our brains and contributes to Alzheimer's plaques that disrupt signals or if the lenses of our eyes become cloudy and we end up with cataracts.

Oxidation forms free radicals, which cause cell death, just like an apple browns when we cut it. Oxidation can be compared to rusting or rotting, and it is a major cause of cellular aging. These processes go on all over our bodies and are responsible for many of the chronic degenerative diseases of aging at its worst extreme, and for the mild aches and pains, mental fog, gastric upset, or other minor maladies that interrupt our well-being.

We can modulate these to a great extent with how, what, and how much we eat. The quality, quantity, and timing of meals can dramatically affect these processes, and slow and perhaps prevent some chronic degenerative diseases of aging.

Quantity Quantified

In the United States, where food is abundant, we supersize our portions. This has created portion distortion. Look at how much things have changed. Twenty years ago a bagel was 3 inches in diameter and 140 calories; today it's 6 inches and 350 calories. Eating a quantity of food that is not being burned as fuel overloads your systems, and excess calories are stored as fat. Sugar binds to protein, and changes the structure and function of those proteins contributing to inflammation and may play a role in cancer development. This is called glycation. Fat is active and releases inflammatory signals that contribute to many disease processes. Here are more examples of how much the size and caloric content of food has changed:

Type	20 years ago	Today
Cookie	1.5 inches; 55 calories	3.5 inches; 275 calories
Caesar Salad	1.5 cups; 390 calories	3.5 cups; 790 calories
Pizza	500 calories	850 calories
Soda	6.5 ounces; 85 calories	20 ounces; 250 calories

Too many calories contributes to obesity and inflammation as well as all of the chronic diseases associated with them. Restricting calories, on the other hand, turns on the longevity genes, and reverses some of the chronic degenerative diseases of aging and the metabolic processes that age us prematurely and cause disease. Eliminate portion distortion for better health and longevity.

Proper Portions

- Meat: 3–4 oz. = the palm of your hand or a deck of cards
- Fish: 3–4 oz. = a checkbook
- Cheese: 1 oz. = 4 dice

- Peanut butter: 2 T. = a ping pong ball
- Pasta: 1 c. = a tennis ball
- Bagel = a hockey puck
- Vegetables: as much as you can hold in 2 hands
- Fruits, grains, milk products: your fist
- Fats and oils: the tip of your thumb

Quality Quest

The quality of the food you eat can turn genes on or off, and cause or reverse glycation, inflammation, and/or oxidation. Whatever you eat builds and repairs your cells, tissues, and organs, or it can damage them. Giving your body the material it needs to function well can dramatically improve your health. Here's an analogy to help you understand why quality is important.

An architect designs specifications for a house and determines the types of materials that will give stability and longevity to the structure to withstand adverse conditions, such as hurricanes, earthquakes, or other natural disasters. If the architect specifies the house should be built with brick, and the suppliers bring a poor-quality wood, the house will be built with whatever you supply. It might not be able to withstand a strong wind and may leak, grow mold, or collapse. Our bodies are built to specifications as well, and we have to be prepared for infection, stress, trauma, and aging.

Hormone levels change as we age (yes, you can control some). Hormones are like project managers that tell cells to regenerate and repair. They coordinate all of the various processes that go on simultaneously in our bodies. Communication occurs through hormones and neurotransmitters. Without the right signaling hormones, if a breakdown occurs, repairs won't take place. This can lead to a weakening of the entire structure. Just imagine the electrical system: A short can cause a malfunction or, if it's big and bad enough, a fire. Using this analogy, and comparing it to food, let's talk about carbohydrates, protein, and fat, otherwise known as macronutrients. This is an oversimplification of the complexity, but, if you understand what happens and how you can influence your metabolism, you can be empowered to take charge of your health.

Glycation: Sugar Browns

Carbohydrates play an important role in modulating insulin and cortisol, which increase as we age. High levels accelerate aging and contribute to degenerative diseases. Consistent high levels of these hormones make them less effective. The term used to describe this is "hormone resistance." When your body becomes resistant to a hormone, it needs higher levels to get the job done.

It takes time to digest and break down a complex carbohydrate, such as whole-grain bread, broccoli, lettuce, or other non-starchy vegetables, so glucose is released slowly and doesn't spike to high levels quickly. Think of a gentle, sloping hill: It rises gradually, it's not steep, and it's not too high. Insulin is made on demand based on the peak of the hill. Insulin is a hormone and is the contractor that tells sugar to go into the cells to be used as fuel or to get stored as fat. The sugar needs a carrier to get it into the cells. If the process happens in a controlled and gradual way using complex carbohydrates, the process runs smoothly. By the time your blood sugar starts to drop, it's time for your next meal. Your blood sugar remains level if it is timed and is released slowly, and if you eat small, frequent meals.

Refined foods, such as white bread, pasta, rice, white foods, sugar, alcohol, or sweetened foods, release sugar quickly, and blood sugar or glucose levels skyrocket. The rise is like a very tall, steep mountain. Insulin, the hormone contractor that directs blood sugar to go into cells or be stored as fat, is made on demand for that very high level of glucose, but its production lags behind. The carriers that are used to get glucose into the cells are overloaded during the spike, so a lot of free glucose circulates. It's like having rogue workers before the contractor arrives, and the excess glucose that can't get carried into the cells to be burned as fuel or stored as fat is free to circulate and bind to proteins all over the body. Just think: It can bind to protein in your brain, forming plaques, and disrupt communication; it can bind to protein in your kidneys and interrupt the filtering process allowing vital nutrients to be filtered out and toxins to remain; it can bind anywhere. This is called glycation.

Receptors are like doormen: They determine what they will let into the cells. They are proteins that respond to signals from hormones like insulin. When insulin levels get too high, the door-men are bombarded with insulin, and just shut the door and don't respond anymore. This is insulin resistance. The receptors resist the signals insulin is sending because they are overloaded. Insulin levels rise because you need more to get a response.

Insulin gives the signal to the receptors to let glucose into cells to be burned as fuel, and what is not immediately needed for energy, insulin directs any excess calories to be stored as fat. When insulin is made for a high level of glucose, because its production lags behind, glucose levels drop fast. This causes low blood glucose, which is a stress on the body. You can get hungry, weak, or light-headed, or get a headache long before its time for your next meal. The low blood glucose drives up cortisol. Cortisol will raise blood sugar, and the whole process continues like a roller-coaster ride. You will read in the next chapter how high levels of cortisol and insulin age us and contribute to inflammatory disease. One of the ways to regulate them is to avoid high spikes in blood sugar.

Avoiding high spikes in blood sugar, along with exercise, a balanced diet, and supplements, keeps your insulin receptors sensitive and responding. Managing stress, which affects your cortisol, is also an important factor in managing blood sugar and insulin, because high cortisol releases blood sugar and the roller-coaster ride continues. Everything in the body is interrelated, so doing only one thing will not necessarily get you the optimal result.

Unload Your Glycemic Load

You can avoid spikes in insulin by eating a low glycemic diet. The glycemic index is the rate at which the blood glucose rises. The glycemic load takes into account the portion size and can predict blood glucose values of different types and amounts of food.

To calculate the glycemic load, multiply the grams of carbohydrate by the glycemic index, and divide by 100.

Glycemic Load = $\dfrac{\text{Grams of carbohydrate X Glycemic Index}}{100}$

The glycemic index uses 50 grams as the standard to compare usable carbohydrate. For example:

- The glycemic index of carrots is about 47.
- Carrots contain about 3.5 grams of carbohydrate per 50g of carrots.

So, to calculate the glycemic load for a standard 50g serving of carrots:

$$\text{GL for carrots} = \frac{3.5 \text{ gm of CHO x GI } 47}{100} = 1.6$$

Lower glycemic index diets reduce blood glucose, triglycerides, weight, and glycation; enhance insulin sensitivity; and improve memory and intellectual performance. Eating a high glycemic diet increases your risk of obesity, type 2 diabetes, high LDL cholesterol, high triglycerides, and cardiovascular diseases such as hardening of the arteries, high blood pressure, heart attack, and stroke. It increases the risk of insulin resistance and metabolic syndrome as well as oxidative stress. Oxidation can destroy your artery walls, damage your DNA, and accelerate inflammation, which is implicated in many of the chronic degenerative diseases of aging.

Know Your Numbers

Measuring your fasting blood sugar is a screening test for diabetes, and hemoglobin A1C can indicate how well controlled your blood sugar is over time. As discussed in Chapter 1, your doctor can measure these through a simple blood test and waist and hip measurements.

- If your fasting blood glucose is high normal, you may be at greater risk of developing diabetes.
- A high hemoglobin A1C can be an indicator that your blood sugar has been elevated long enough to glycate proteins.
- An elevated fasting insulin level can be a sign of insulin resistance.
- A waist-to-hip ratio in women greater than 0.80, and in men greater than 0.90, is a fairly accurate predictor of an

increased risk of obesity-related conditions and of increased risk of cardiovascular disease and diabetes.

	Fasting Blood Sugar (in milligrams per deciliters)	Hemoglobin A1C (HbA1C)	Fasting Insulin Units iUI/ml
Ideal	65–86 mg/dl	< 5%	<6 iUI/ml
Normal	<100 mg/dl	< 6%	6-27 iUI/ml
Pre-diabetes	100–125 mg/dl	>6%	>15 Insulin Resistance
Diabetes	> 126 mg/dl	> 7%	

Compiled and adapted from "A Comprehensive Guide to Preventive Blood Testing" (**Life Extension Magazine,** May 2004), and "Aging and Glycation" (**Life Extension Magazine,** April 2008).

Eating a low glycemic diet can decrease the risk of developing disease, and can actually reverse some of the negative effects of high blood sugar and enable you to reduce or eliminate medication. You can also slow the absorption of sugar by combing it with fiber, protein, and fat.

Glycemic Index and Load

	Glycemic Index	Glycemic Load	Examples
Low	< 55	< 10	Most fruits, vegetables, whole grains, legumes, chicken, fish, nuts, fructose
Medium	56–69	11–19	Whole wheat, basmati rice, sweet potatoes, sucrose
High	> 70	> 20	White bread, white rice, potatoes, watermelon, many breakfast cereals, glucose

Compiled and adapted from the International Table of Glycemic Index and Glycemic Load Values: 2002 from *The American Journal of Clinical Nutrition.*

Good resources for determining the food with low glycemic

index or glycemic load are the Harvard Publications website ("Glycemic index and glycemic load for 100+ foods") and the book *The Glyceminc Load Counter.* (See the References.)

Eating a low glycemic diet and timing your meals to keep blood sugar levels even are important in reversing or preventing cardiovascular disease, obesity, type 2 diabetes, lipid disorders, inflammation, and oxidation, which plays a role in many other illnesses.

Oxidation: Rust Less

Oxidation occurs naturally in all of our cells. It is a by-product of energy production. Eating, breathing, and exercising produce free radicals that oxidize, or rust, our cells and, without antioxidant support, these free radicals cause oxidation, inflammation, and cell death. Inflammation speeds up oxidation, and oxidation produces inflammation. Colorful foods are rich in antioxidants that capture free radicals.

Eating a variety of colors in your fruits and vegetables will give you a variety of antioxidants, along with green tea, and herbs and spices. The highest antioxidant levels are found in clove, followed by allspice, oregano, sage, cinnamon, peppermint, rosemary, thyme, marjoram, ginger, mustard, garlic, and coriander. Some also have anti-inflammatory properties and other medicinal effects, so eat a variety of all colors of fruits and vegetables, and spice up your life to age-less.

Tips for choosing carbohydrate:

- Eat a low glycemic diet (foods with a glycemic load of less than 9, ideally less than 7).

- Eat complex carbohydrates high in fiber, especially vegetables.

- Avoid highly processed foods.

- Limit sugar, starch, starchy vegetables, and white foods such as bread, pasta, rice, potatoes, and sugar.

- Eat small frequent meals every four to five hours.

- To slow the rise in blood sugar, combine carbohydrates

with some protein and fat.

- Avoid sugary soft drinks and cereals.
- Eat a rainbow of colors and add a variety of herbs and spices.

Put Out the Fire: Fat Facts

Fats are essential to our health. They do so much more than add to your waistline. Fatty acids, the building blocks of fat, perform many functions, such as the following:

- Source of energy and hormone production
- Structural components for cells
- Regulates gene expression for lipid, carbohydrate, and protein metabolism
- Regulates cell growth and differentiation (the ability to change a stem cell into other types of cells)
- Provides insulation and temperature regulation
- Protects our joints and organs

Eicosanoids are made from fatty acids and act as signaling molecules, telling your body how to respond. They act as hormones and serve as communicators to our cells and organ systems to regulate inflammation, cellular function, mood, and behavior.

Eicosanoids can be inflammatory or anti-inflammatory. What you eat determines this balance. You need inflammation to fight infection and repair damage; however, an overabundance of inflammation is implicated in inflammatory diseases such as allergy, asthma, arthritis, Alzheimer's, autoimmune disease, cancer, and more. The balance of Omega 6 to Omega 3 fatty acids is what determines which signal you will make — inflammation or anti-inflammation — and this is determined by your diet.

What we eat has changed a lot. In Paleolithic (prehistoric) times our diets were mostly plant-based, and the ratio of Omega 6 to Omega 3 fatty acids was 1:1 or 2:1. This ratio was perfect for balancing the inflammatory response and preventing chronic inflammatory diseases. Our Western diets have a ratio of 10:1

to 25:1, and are considered inflammatory. Changing the ratio of Omega 6 to Omega 3 is very important in reversing or preventing these and other types of diseases. Studies have shown that changing the ratio can prevent or modulate disease. Here are some examples:

- 4:1 was associated with a 70% decrease in total mortality from cardiovascular disease.

- 2.5:1 reduced rectal cancer cell growth in patients with colorectal cancer.

- 2-3:1 suppressed inflammation in patients with rheumatoid arthritis.

- 5:1 had a beneficial effect on patients with asthma.

- The lower Omega 6 to Omega 3 ratio in women with breast cancer was associated with decreased risk.

This chart is a generalization of how to determine if a fat has inflammatory or anti-inflammatory properties and which foods have more Omega 6 or Omega 3 fatty acids.

Omega 6	Omega 3
Generally inflammatory	Generally anti-inflammatory
Solid at room temperature	Liquid at room temperature
Meat, eggs, dairy; arachidonic acid	Olive and canola oil, avocado, nuts (walnuts, almonds, macadamia)
Some are anti-inflammatory, such as flax, borage, grapeseed, and primrose oil	Cold-water fish (mackerel, salmon, tuna, herring)
Inflammatory eicosanoids	Anti-inflammatory eicosanoids

Fish oil has many types of fatty acids. However, the Eicosapentaenoic acid (EPA) and Docosahexaenoic acid (DHA) components are the fatty acids that have been shown to reduce inflammation and have been used to improve many illnesses. Studies using EPA/DHA in fish oil have shown improvements in depression, bipolar disorders, mood, ADHD, and schizophrenia, and may hold promise for other inflammatory disorders such as Alzheimer's, cancer, cardiovascular disease, rheumatoid arthritis, osteoporosis, and asthma, as well as spinal cord and traumatic brain injury.

Many of my patients balk at the thought of swallowing more than one fish oil capsule. Just think: If your ratio is 10:1 or 25:1 of Omega 6 to Omega 3 fatty acids, and you need to change that balance, you will need more than you can get in fish alone. In general, most high-potency fish oil capsules are approximately 0.7 grams.

Food	Grams of fat
Fish oil capsule	0.7
Flounder filet, baked (4 oz.)	2.1
Chicken breast, skinned, roasted (4 oz.)	4.8
Sirloin steak, broiled (4 oz.)	5.4
Extra-lean (95%) beef burger, broiled (4 oz.)	7.4
Regular beef burger (4 oz.)	22.3
Medium fries	20

Source: NutriBase: U.S. Department of Agriculture database.

This is why I recommend taking fish oil. Be sure to look at the EPA/DHA content, since these are the components we are looking for. Some fish oils have other fats and may have a higher gram content but do not have the high levels of EPA/DHA that we need to lower our Omega 6 to Omega 3 ratio. When buying a fish oil, add up the EPA and DHA milligrams to determine how much active anti-inflammatory activity your fish oil has. Most people need 1,000–2,000 milligrams.

Rebuilding a healthier body with quality fat takes time. Just as you renovate a house brick by brick, this takes time and patience. Since our cells turn over and we are continually producing hormones and cell-signaling molecules made from whatever fat we give our bodies, it will take time before you reverse the ratio. However, you will get many benefits fairly quickly that will build over time.

Tips for choosing fat and to restore Omega 6 to Omega 3 balance:

- Decrease the amount of saturated fats in your diet, such as meat and dairy.

- Avoid trans fats, saturated fats, and hydrogenated oils. Read labels.

- Eat meat from animals that have been grass-fed. Grain-fed meats have more Omega 6 and grass-fed have more Omega 3 fatty acids.

- Eat fish with a high Omega 3 content, such as mackerel, tuna, herring, and salmon.

- Eat nuts and oils high in anti-inflammatory fatty acids such as olive, canola, avocado, walnuts, almonds, and macadamia nuts.

- Take at least 1–2 grams of EPA/DHA found in fish oil. You may need more depending on your condition. However, seek the advice of your doctor, since high levels may interfere with medication and thin your blood.

Protein Package

Protein is required for growth, to repair damaged cells and tissue, to make hormones, and for a variety of other metabolic activities. There are several things you need to know about proteins.

- Eat a variety of protein sources to assure you are getting all of the essential amino acids.

- Learn what proteins are combined with. Proteins in food are either combined with carbohydrate or fat.

- Food allergies are caused by the protein component of food.

- There is a difference between food allergy, intolerance, and sensitivity.

Proteins are made up of amino acids. Some are essential because your body cannot make them, and we must get them from outside sources in our diet. Others are non-essential because they can be produced in our body. There are multiple sources of proteins available; however, animal sources of protein contain all essential amino acids and are considered complete sources of protein, whereas plant proteins lack some of the essential amino acids and are therefore classified as incomplete. Combining plant proteins will enable you to get all of the essential amino acids. It is important to eat a variety of food to get all of the amino acids you need.

Protein in food is usually mixed with carbohydrate or fat. As we discussed above, the type and balance of fat can modulate inflammation. Choosing chicken and fish as your main sources of protein can improve your Omega 6 to Omega 3 ratio. Beans are a very good source of incomplete protein and are packed with carbohydrate and fiber, but they must be combined with other plant proteins to get all of the essential amino acids.

It is the protein component of food that causes allergic reactions. The most common food allergies are milk, eggs, peanuts, tree nuts (almonds, cashews, walnuts), fish (bass, cod, flounder), shellfish (lobster, crab, shrimp), wheat, and soy.

Food Allergy, Intolerance, and Sensitivity

Some people have intolerances to food, which are different from allergies. Gluten is a protein that occurs in grains such as wheat, barley, and rye. Gluten sensitivity is common, and can cause a serious reaction in people who have celiac disease, a digestive disorder. However, some people never develop full-blown celiac disease and may have gluten intolerance. Gluten has been implicated in autoimmune diseases such as thyroiditis, multiple sclerosis, and ulcerative colitis, and can cause vague symptoms in some people. Many cases are now detected in adulthood during investigation of problems as diverse as anemia, osteoporosis, autoimmune disorders, unexplained neurological syndromes, and infertility. More cardiovascular disease has been found in patients with autoimmune disease. The incidence of cardiovascular disease in various autoimmune disorders is increased 10- to 30-fold in comparison to the general population.

Intolerances may be caused by a deficiency of an enzyme necessary to break down or process a food component. Lactose intolerance is a concern for the majority of the world's population due to low levels of lactase, an enzyme that breaks down lactose in milk. Histamine intolerance can occur in people who have low levels of diamine oxidase. Fish, cheese, hard cured sausages, pickled cabbage, and alcoholic beverages can contain histamine. Intolerances can occur to other foods, additives and preservatives, coloring, emulsifiers and taste enhancers, and toxins. Intolerance can also develop to foods that are not fully digested or absorbed. Intolerances cause symptoms ranging from headache, gas, bloating, joint aches, nasal congestion, mucous, fatigue, or other symptoms. These may not be true allergies. However, the best way to determine if you have food intolerances is to do an elimination diet using supportive nutrients and herbs that detoxify and cleanse.

Elimination Diet

An elimination diet removes all of the common allergens and foods that are most likely to cause intolerance, as well as dyes, preservatives, and artificial ingredients. The elimination process can assist in overcoming food addiction and unmasking problem foods so that you can associate cause and effect. It can be an important tool for diagnosing food intolerances and allergies, as well as allowing you to quiet inflammation and to heal. Most people feel renewed energy and vitality after the first week. Introducing a new food every three days and observing symptoms can uncover hidden food intolerances and avoiding that food can give relief from symptoms. (Instructions for how to do an elimination diet are in Appendix IV.)

Diets high in lean protein can improve weight and fat loss as well as lowering triglycerides, improving blood sugar control and insulin sensitivity, and lowering C reactive protein, a biomarker of inflammation.

Tips for choosing protein:

- Eat a variety of food to assure you are getting all of the essential amino acids.
- Trim fat from meats and poultry. Grill, broil, or bake meats and poultry, and avoid frying.

- Choose lean protein such as beans and fish as well as low-fat dairy.
- Balance your protein, carbohydrate, and fat.
- Avoid foods that cause symptoms of allergy or intolerance.

Eat to Live

A longevity diet is low in calories yet is packed with nutrients, especially with regard to phytonutrients in the form of antioxidants and flavonoids found in all of the colored fruits and vegetables. Research suggests that diets associated with a reduced risk of chronic diseases are vegetable- and fruit-heavy (therefore phytonutrient-rich and antioxidant-rich) but reduced in meat, refined grains, saturated fat, sugar, salt, and full-fat dairy products. The low levels of saturated fat, high antioxidant intake, and low glycemic load in these diets are likely contributing to a decreased risk for cardiovascular disease, some cancers, and other chronic diseases through multiple mechanisms, including reduced oxidative stress.

Some ABCs of Weight Maintenance

Since obesity is an epidemic and a major contributor to the chronic degenerative diseases of aging, here are some tips to trim your waistline and shed those pounds.

Attitude is everything: When you crave something, oftentimes it's not because you are hungry, but because you are stressed, bored, anxious, or just thinking about something and want it. Recognizing your triggers is the first step, then asking yourself if you are truly hungry. If you are hungry, choose a healthy option. If you are not hungry, distract yourself with a pleasurable activity. Avoid using food as a reward. Plan how you will respond in social situations when there is pressure to eat larger quantities or make unhealthy choices. If your cravings, impulses, and food addictions are more difficult to overcome, a coach or therapist can assist you.

Balance protein, carbohydrates, and fats at every meal: Controlling the digestion and release of carbohydrates will enable you to manage spikes of cortisol and insulin, which store fat, especially in your midsection. A 40% carbohydrate, 30% protein, and 30% fat ratio of calories is best for managing the insulin response. An active person may need to increase the carbohydrates. Combining protein, carbohydrate, and fat acts to release carbohydrates more slowly. An easy way to look at this is to divide your plate into thirds:

- 2/3 of your plate should be non-starchy vegetables.
  - o Fruit is half the amount of vegetables.
  - o Starchy vegetable servings are half a vegetable serving. Grains fit in this category.
- 1/3 of your plate should be lean protein (chicken; fish; lean, grass-fed, organic beef; beans; protein isolates).
- Fat should be a condiment. (Sprinkle oil, cheese, avocado, olives, or nuts.)

Choose healthier proteins, carbohydrates, and fats: The type or quality of protein, carbohydrate, and fat can make a big difference in optimizing your health.

Delight in activities that don't involve food: Choose pleasurable activities as a reward, and look at food choices as fuel. Discover new recipes that are healthy, satisfying, and enjoyable.

Eat every four hours: This will help to reduce hunger and keep blood sugar levels stable. Snacks such as fruit and nuts, hummus, and vegetables can curb your appetite and keep blood sugar level.

Fitness is fundamental: Walking is the easiest way to get aerobic activity. Work your way up to 10,000 steps per day, or do some form of aerobic activity and resistance training. The new American College of Sports Medicine and American Heart Association Guidelines are five days a week of moderate intensity cardiovascular activities and two additional days of strength training. The duration varies according to your goal, as follows:

- General health benefits: 30 minutes
- Avoid weight gain: 30–50 minutes
- Weight loss: 45–84 minutes
- Prevent weight regain after loss: 40–60 minutes

Work on strength, endurance, flexibility, and balance, for overall health. Interval training is a great way to burn calories and build cardiopulmonary fitness. However, be sure you are conditioned and start slow with very short intervals.

Glycemic index: Eat a low glycemic diet and decrease your daily intake of sugar.

- For weight loss on a 1,200-calorie diet:
  - Eat no more than 15–45 grams of sugar per day. The lower end is better to decrease the insulin response.
  - Eat no more than 120 grams of carbohydrate a day.
- For weight loss on a 1,500-calorie diet:
  - Eat no more than 15–59 grams of sugar per day. The lower end is better to decrease the insulin response.
  - Eat no more than 150 grams of carbohydrate a day.

Have a healthy portion: Follow the portion sizes recommended in this chapter, and add more if you are doing strenuous activity

Ingest supplements: Supplements help to manage dietary deficiencies, inflammation, cravings, and fat burning. A good multivitamin, magnesium, fish oil, Hoodia gordonii, bitter orange, fucoxanthin, L carnitine, and conjugated linoleic acid are some of the supplements that can aid weight loss. Talk to your doctor about what is appropriate for you.

Success Stories

Let's look how some dietary changes helped Nan and Ernest.

Nan's diet consisted of a lot of whole grains, fruit, and poultry, and did not have a lot of vegetables. Her portion sizes were good, and she timed her meals correctly. She did an elimination diet and used products with detoxifying nutrients and herbs. She lost 6 pounds, she felt alert and clear, and her energy was restored. She noted that once she added non-organic poultry or meats into her diet or processed foods with additives or preservatives, the symptoms returned. She was able to eat organic, non-antibiotic, hormone-free meats and poultry. We concluded that it was possible that she reacted to traces of antibiotics and hormones that were in the meat and possibly some food additives. She took a multivitamin, fish oil, probiotics, and digestive enzymes; only ate meat and poultry that were organic; and added more vegetables to her diet; and she felt so much better. Her clarity and energy returned, and she was better able to lose weight.

Ernest hardly ate throughout the day. He saved his big meal for the evening and was famished. The portions he ate were large, and his diet was very high in refined carbohydrate and saturated fat. He also did an elimination diet, and his minor aches and pains disappeared. He felt light and clear. He found that wheat and dairy products made him tired and achy, and contributed to his lack of energy and focus. He followed a Mediterranean-style diet, shortened the time between meals by having healthy snacks of berries and nuts or hummus and vegetables, and limited the amount of red meat, wheat, and dairy he ate. He continued to lose weight; started a balanced exercise program; took a multivitamin, high-dose fish oil and magnesium, niacin, nattokinase, and other supplements; and was able to stop his medication for blood pressure and cholesterol control. His sex life improved, and he feels like he did as a young man.

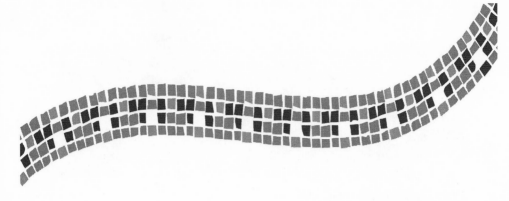

Chapter 3
Supplement Savvy

Can You Relate?

Do you have fatigue, diabetes, high cholesterol, or high blood pressure? Are you having trouble with memory, depression, or sleep? Could supplements help or harm you?

Katrina, a 23-year-old, was taking an over-the-counter herbal preparation. She applied for a job and tested positive on her drug test. As a Medical Review Officer, I believed her story and asked her to bring in the supplement. I sent it to our lab, and it had high quantities of a benzodiazepine, an anxiety-reducing drug in it. The ingredients on the label were disguised.

Paul, a 52-year-old who complained of dry eyes, brought the expensive primrose oil to a colleague of mine because it wasn't helping him. My colleague sent it to a laboratory to be tested. He told Paul it would help, but it was not the brand he recommended. The results showed that, although the product claimed to have 100% primrose oil in it, there was less than 5% primrose oil; the rest was cheap canola oil.

Mark, a 45-year-old owner of a mid-sized company, married with three children, led a high-stress life. He complained of anxiety, fatigue, and mental fog. His symptoms made him irritable, and he was getting worried because his irritability affected his relationship with his wife and children, and the mental fog affected his decision-making. He was taking an over-the-counter stress formula and also one for memory that was recommended by someone in a health food store. However, he didn't feel any different.

Ann, mother of three and co-owner of a business, had a significant amount of stress and anxiety. She wasn't sleeping well and had outbursts of anger and irritability followed by depression. Her relationships were being affected, and she was embarrassed by her behavior. She was taking some herbs and a stress vitamin formula recommended by a nutritionist and didn't feel they were helping her.

I was trained in a traditional way and was not a big believer in supplements. I studied a lot about nutrition during my college years, and then I dabbled in it when I was in medical school and residency. The more I read studies in scientific journals, the more I realized there is some validity to them. It made sense, and I started to suggest that my patients take some supplements for various conditions and saw them benefit. The *New England Journal of Medicine,* one of the most prestigious and highly regarded medical journals, published on January 2, 1992, an article stating that one in three people sought some alternative care. A 1998 study showed that the use of alternative medicine had risen from 33.8% in 1990 to 42.1% in 1997. Since that was a large number, I felt that I should know more about some of the things my patients were doing, and I don't do many things superficially. I read extensively, took classes, and studied under some experts in their fields. Supplements became a part of my treatment regime, along with standard pharmaceuticals and lifestyle guidelines.

Deficiencies Are Common

Analyzing people's diets in a computerized program and running metabolic and micronutrient tests made me a believer. I saw deficiencies that affected people's health. I did more research for a talk and discovered that the global populations and U.S. have many dietary nutritional deficiencies. These are widespread and global, they range from childhood to the elderly, and they affect affluent as well as impoverished people. Here are some excerpts of what I found from the studies:

- The Center for Nutrition Policy and Promotion conducted a survey in 2005 called the Healthy Eating Index and looked at the number of servings of food categories consumed. Scores were 48% below requirements for everything except grains, meat, and beans, and were less than half for dark green and orange vegetables, legumes, and whole grains.

- The U.S. Department of Health and Human Services and U.S. Department of Agriculture Dietary Guidelines for Americans 2005 found that the following nutrients may be low enough to be of concern for adults: calcium, potassium, fiber, magnesium, and Vitamins A (as carotenoids), C, and E.

- A study of two U.S. populations found nutritional deficits of Vitamin A, E, folic acid, potassium, and calcium that were very low, and marginally low for Vitamin C and some B vitamins. They concluded that most elderly U.S. citizens were likely to be deficient in five micronutrients and marginally insufficient in four others.

Studies like these were conducted all over the world, and nutritional deficiencies were prevalent on most continents and in a variety of socioeconomic and age groups.

Vitamin D

I've also read the medical literature and many Web-based news articles. Over the past two years a lot has been written about Vitamin

D, which is actually a hormone. The amount of information on Vitamin D deficiency is astounding. It affects more than half the adults in the world. The National Health and Nutrition Examination Survey (NHANES) found data demonstrating a marked decrease in Vitamin D levels from the 1988–1994 to the 2001–2004 NHANES data collections. The conclusion was that current recommendations for Vitamin D supplementation are inadequate to address the growing epidemic of Vitamin D insufficiency.

Here are some statistics on the percentages of people with Vitamin D deficiency:

- 36% of healthy adults aged 18–29
- 40% of adults in sunny Miami during the winter
- 57% of the general U.S. population
- The majority of the elderly

Still not convinced that many of us, even the health-conscious who eat right and take supplements, can be deficient? I enter what my patients eat into a nutritional analysis program using the data on food labels and the nutritional content of foods from a database from the U.S. Department of Agriculture. It confirms much of what this data suggests: We do not have enough nutrients in our food. Nutrients may be lost by not picking the food fully ripened. Nutrients are lost in shipping and storage, and they are lost in cooking. So what's left by the time we eat it? All of them are not fully absorbed, and everything may not get into your cells or do what they are supposed to do when they get in there.

Does a Multi a Day Keep the Doctor Away?

Many of my patients take a multivitamin. I do, too. Multivitamins are the most popular dietary supplements. People have a false sense of security when taking them. They don't realize that some contain ingredients that are not well -absorbed or synthetic versions of some vitamins, which may actually have deleterious effects. The ingredients vary widely by brand, and it is difficult to know whether a company adheres to good manufacturing processes used to assure quality, potency, and purity.

There are no established standards on what multivitamins should contain. One reason for not having uniform standards is that people's diets and their needs differ. Nutrient requirements and cautions vary depending on age, gender, and health status, use of substances such as alcohol or tobacco, and medications taken.

A lot of complexity and confusion exist regarding supplements, and we are all continuing to learn more and more. Some reasons you may not be getting benefits from supplements include:

- Poor quality

- Inadequate dose

- Form not beneficial

- Combination is missing something

- Poor absorption

- Poor assimilation (getting into the cells and doing its job)

Quality Counts

You saw from the cases I wrote about at the beginning of the chapter that supplements can contain unwanted contaminants and/or are worthless because of little or no active ingredients, so buyer beware. I follow reports in health newsletters and watchdog organizations that test supplements. Many well-known brands do not have the potency or purity stated on their labels. This is why I suggest buying brands that manufacture under the strictest FDA guidelines, known as "pharmaceutical or clinical grade." These companies use Good Manufacturing Processes (GMP). They test what is going into their products for potency and purity, and they assure consumers that there is no contamination throughout the manufacturing process. Many have control over the process, and own and operate their own plants. Be certain that the company whose brand you buy uses an independent company to certify its potency and purity. Some companies perform research studies using their products to determine if they benefit people with certain conditions. Quality and quality control are important. There are consumer organizations such as Consumer Lab that monitor supplements (consumerlab.com). You can always ask the manufacturer if they use a third party to test their products and obtain a certificate of analysis.

Dose and Form Make a Difference

Many of my patients comment that they tried one supplement or another and it didn't work. I look at what they are taking and find that sometimes they are not taking the right dose, the right form, or the right combination for their particular problems and needs. We can do trial and error to determine all of that, or do metabolic, genetic single nucleotide polymorphism (SNP) testing and/ or micronutrient testing to come up with a formula that is specific to their unique genetic, metabolic, and nutritional profile.

You may want to look at it like this: If you have a plant and only give it water and not enough sunlight, it may survive but not thrive. If you then give it enough water and sunlight but plant it in a soil that is too acidic or not appropriate for that particular type of plant, the same thing may happen: The plant may live, but it might not thrive. The same is true of a supplement regimen. It's rarely one thing. A higher dose of one supplement may become toxic. It's a unique combination of many components, at the right dose, and in the right form that will allow a person to absorb supplements, correct deficiencies, and bypass metabolic blocks to create energy, repair and regenerate tissue, and achieve optimum function. To gain a better understanding of metabolism and testing refer to Chapter 7.

It would take an entire book dedicated to vitamins and minerals and volumes of references to make a solid case for why someone may need supplements and/or higher doses of supplements. Here's the rationale as to why you would consider taking supplements.

- You can see that a government agency has determined almost half the population is deficient in certain nutrients.

- We know that nutritional deficiencies can cause illness.

- What is most controversial is what is optimal, not just the bare minimum.

- Would it make sense to you if you have an illness that may be associated with a nutritional deficiency or are taking a medication that may deplete certain nutrients to look there first?

I don't believe in an either-or mentality. I believe in using what is most effective with the least amount of risk. The recommended daily allowance, or RDA, of a nutrient is based on the amount needed to prevent a deficiency. It was developed for populations, not individuals. The bare minimum may not be what is optimal. Optimal is when you are not on the brink of developing disease. Optimal is when your body gets what it needs to function and to deal with the onslaught of physical, emotional, and environmental stressors, or speed genetic enzyme variations or bypass metabolic blocks. Optimal is having a reserve. If you are deficient in a nutrient, you may need more than the RDA, because you not only have to meet your minimum requirements; you have to correct the deficiency.

If we just look at the most common deficiencies cited in the literature, and look at the nutrient content for those in some popular over-the-counter (OTC) multivitamins (MVA) and compare to the doses used in studies that showed benefit from their use, we see the dosages that were used in the studies to show benefit were much higher than that found in a typical over-the-counter multivitamin as follows:

Nutrient	OTC MVA	OTC% RDA	Dosages Used in Studies
Vitamin A	2500–3500 IU	50–70	100,000 IU+
Magnesium	50–100 mg	13–25	250 mg+
Calcium	210–500 mg	21–25	500 mg+
Folate	200–400 mcg	50–100	500 mcg+
Vitamin E	22.5–45 IU	75–150	100 IU+
Fiber	0	0	25 gm

Fiber is not a component of multivitamins and while it is generally found in fruits, vegetables, grains, and legumes, diets high in processed foods do not supply enough, and a supplement may be warranted.

Better Form, Better Function

The form of the vitamin can make a big difference: natural versus synthetic, single or mixed, oxide or amino acid chelate. One's head can spin with all the variations seen in a health food store. Some companies choose a supplement form based on its widespread use, others because the compound is less bulky (that is, people need fewer pills to get the desired dose), and others choose a form based on cost.

To go through every vitamin and its form is beyond the scope of this book. Therefore we will look at the forms of nutrients that are most often deficient.

- **Vitamin A:** Vitamin A is really a group of compounds: preformed Vitamin A and carotenoids. Vitamin A usually refers to its preformed or retinol form (including retinyl palmitate and retinyl acetate) found in animal products such as eggs, milk, and liver. Provitamin A, found in colorful fruits and vegetables, has a well-known carotenoid called Beta-carotene; it is converted in the body to vitamin A based on the body's need for Vitamin A. Of the 563 identified carotenoids, fewer than 10% can be made into Vitamin A in the body. Lycopene, lutein, and zeaxanthin are carotenoids that do not have Vitamin A activity but have other health-promoting properties. It is best to choose a combination of natural, full-spectrum mixed carotenoids Vitamin A, since each has a specific beneficial effect. Keep in mind that some studies that showed harmful effects used the synthetic forms. Vitamin A palmitate is best for people who have trouble absorbing fats.

- **Magnesium:** Magnesium oxide is found most frequently in supplements since it is less bulky, and a consumer would find that fewer pills are necessary to get the desired dose. However, magnesium oxide is not as well absorbed as other forms. Magnesium citrate, on the other hand, is very well absorbed; however, in high doses it can cause diarrhea. This would work well in someone who was constipated, but if someone needed a high dose and developed diarrhea, I would use magnesium glycinate, which is well absorbed and has less effect on the GI tract.

- **Calcium:** Calcium citrate, malate, and hydroxyapatite are the most absorbable forms. The bioavailabilty of calcium citrate is 2.5 times that of calcium carbonate, the most commonly used form. You can only absorb 500 mg at one time, so split the dose if you take more than 500mg.

- **Folate:** Folate occurs naturally in foods in different forms such as tetrahydrofolate, 5-methyltetrahydrofolate, 5 formyltetrahydrofolate (folinic acid), and others. Folic acid is its synthetic (man-made) form. Some people cannot transform folate into its active form or change it to the other methyl forms. Some people need the 5 formyl tetrahydrofolate form (5- formyl THF) or the 5 –methyl tetrahydrofolate (5-MTHF) form. Otherwise folate is a good form of this vitamin. If taking a folic acid supplement, do not exceed 400 mcg, because you can mask a Vitamin B 12 deficiency, and many foods are fortified with folic acid.

- **Vitamin E:** The most common form found in supplements is alpha tocopherol. However, natural Vitamin E, gamma tocopherol, is the most absorbable and potent form. Mixed tocopherols are the most complete. Vitamin E succinate is a dry, oil-free powder form that is good for people who have trouble absorbing fat.

- **Fiber:** Dietary fiber is the indigestible part of plants and has two forms: soluble fiber and insoluble fiber. Soluble fiber is important, since it is a source of food for the good bacteria in the gut, which ferments it, and produces vitamins such as biotin and Vitamin K and beneficial short chain fatty acids that are important for gut health. It also binds to bile acids and removes steroid hormones and cholesterol. It is found in beans, oat bran, barley, rye, apples, prunes, plums, and berries. Insoluble fiber is otherwise known as roughage. It absorbs excess fluids from the bowel and stimulates bowel movements. It is mostly found in whole grains, nuts, and seeds. If you are looking for a supplement, look for ingredients such as psyllium, beta glucan, fructo oligosaccharides (FOS), acacia gum, guar gum, inulin, apple pectin, psyllium husk, flax, prune, or the terms dietary and soluble fiber.

- **EPA/DHA Fish Oil**: Look for the EPA/DHA content. Because Omega 3 fatty acids are obtained from natural sources, levels in supplements can vary, depending on the source and method of processing. The EPA and DHA content in the pills and liquids can vary by as much as 10-fold. Concentration depends on the source of the Omega 3s, how the oil is processed, and the amounts of other ingredients included in the supplement. Purchase fish oil products certified as free of significant levels of mercury, toxic organochlorines, and PCBs. Fish oil can thin the blood, so if you have a bleeding disorder or you are on blood thinners, consult your doctor.

Choosing a Supplement Regimen

I often get asked what a good supplement regimen is, and it's a hard question to answer for the general public. I do customized, personalized medicine. A good place to start is to choose the highest-quality supplements from a reputable company, tested by an independent third party that adheres to the highest standards of quality control called pharmaceutical or clinical grade.

If you are healthy and have no issues, consider taking the following:
- Multivitamin and mineral formula
- EPA/DHA fish oil — 1,000–2,000 mg of the EPA +DHA component (more if you have an inflammatory disease)
- Vitamin D_3 — 1,000–2,000 IU (measure levels; you may need more or less)
- A probiotic of 10–25 billion cfu units especially if you have allergies, asthma, or autoimmune disease, which may

require much higher doses

- Calcium citrate or hydroxyapetite — 500–1,000 mg if not enough in your multivitamin; the dose will depend on your age, sex, and pregnancy status, as well as dietary intake.

Multivitamin (MVA) Guidelines

Your needs will vary based on age, sex, medications you take, and other conditions. A perfectly healthy young person could start on the low end of the scale, and an older person on many medications may lean toward the higher end. These are conservative doses. Be sure to check with your doctor for interactions with medication or medical conditions, especially if you have liver or kidney disease.

Vitamin	Dose	Mineral	Dose
Vitamin A*	5–15,000 IU	Boron	0.25–3 mg
Mixed carotenoids	11–25,000 mg	Calcium	100–600 mg
Vitamin B complex B1,2,3,6	25–100 mg	Chromium	200–500 mcg
Vitamin B12	25–1,000 mcg	Copper	1–3 mg
Vitamin C	500–2,000 mg		
Vitamin D	200–1,000 IU	Magnesium	400–600 mg
Vitamin E Mixed tocopherols	200–400 IU	Manganese	2.5–5 mg
Biotin	300–1,000 mg	Molybdenum	50–200mcg
Choline	25–100 mg	Potassium	25–100 mg
Folic Acid	400–800 mcg	Selenium	100–300 mcg
PABA	25–500 mg	Vanadium	30-200 mcg
Pantothenic acid	25–400 mg	Zinc	10–30 mg

*Note: Smokers should not use more than 8,000 IU of Vitamin A.

You Are Unique

If you have health concerns, are on medications, or are looking to vitamins and supplements to modulate disease or risk factors, it's best to work with a knowledgeable healthcare practitioner to determine the best combination for you. Functional tests are available to determine your nutritional status and absorption of vitamins into your bloodstream, and some can determine if they are actually getting into your cells and working. You can also have metabolic or genetic tests to determine your unique needs. Seek the advice of a health care professional who is well versed in this arena.

Let's look at how supplement choices affected Katrina, Paul, Mark, and Ann from the beginning of the chapter.

Success Stories

Katrina was cleared for her job and was told about the benzodiazepine in the supplement she was taking. She was advised to seek medical care and practice stress-reduction techniques. We educated her regarding choosing supplements and advised her to use pharmaceutical-grade products that were third-party tested.

Paul was told that the supplement he was taking had little to no primrose oil, which was the active ingredient necessary to help his condition. He was advised to take a pharmaceutical-grade formula that was more expensive, and his symptoms improved.

Mark eliminated processed foods, cut down on sugar, refined carbohydrates, caffeine, and alcohol, and was prescribed high dose pharmaceutical-grade B 50 complex, Vitamin C, magnesium, fish oil, and calming herbs such as valerian, passion–flower, and hops. He still didn't respond well, so we did metabolic testing. He was low in amino acids and neurotransmitters, so we supplemented with 5-hydroxytryptophan (5 HTP), GABA, methionine, and taurine, and we stopped the calming herbs. He did not follow a good diet initially, but once he started to feel better and get a good night's sleep, he began to exercise and eat better. His anxiety abated, he felt more sure of himself, and he became calm and clear. His wife was very pleased with his progress.

Ann eliminated processed foods and cut down on sugar, refined carbohydrates, caffeine, and alcohol. She still had regular periods, was ovulating, and had adequate progesterone. However, her estrogen levels were high in relation to her progesterone. She was prescribed high dose pharmaceutical-grade B 50 complex, Vitamin C, magnesium, fish oil, and calming herbs such as valerian, passion-flower, and hops as well as soluble fiber and indole-3-carbinol. She did extremely well and no longer had outbursts of anger and irritability.

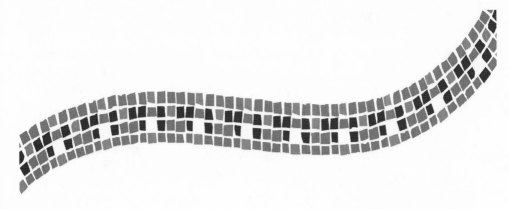

Chapter 4
Be FIT — BE SaFE

Can You Relate?

A re you stiff and sore, tired and achy? Or are you weak, unable to open a jar, or not able to climb stairs as well as you used to? Is your memory poor, or are you depressed? If you have tight clothing, a weight problem, diabetes, osteoporosis, or a whole host of other problems, there is a lot you can do. One major component of managing these is exercise.

> Martha walks every day and does a lot of lifting, and considers herself to be strong and fit. She slipped, lost her balance, and fractured her wrist. Testing revealed poor balance, loss of handgrip strength even in her non-fractured hand, mild bone loss called osteopenia, and high cholesterol.
>
> Jim likes to lift weights in the gym several times a week, and suffered a rotator cuff tear and tendonitis in his elbow. Testing revealed good overall strength and, no surprise, a lack of flexibility and endurance.

What Martha and Jim have in common are exercise routines that are not well balanced. Why is this important? We are learning that the reasons why exercise is so important is it helps us avoid injury, keeps our bodies fit and strong, gets circulation to all of our body parts, preserves our heart, lung, brain, and kidney function, helps us maintain mobility, and more. However to truly meet these goals and to age gracefully and healthfully, having all the components for fitness can help us accomplish these goals.

Exercise to BE SaFE

Balance

Hip fractures can land you in the hospital and nursing home. The American Academy of Orthopedic Surgeons noted on their website, "Most hip fracture patients who previously lived independently will require assistance from their family or home care. Forty percent of hip fracture patients 65 and older are discharged or transferred from hospitals to long-term care facilities. All hip fracture patients require walking aids for several months after injury, and nearly half will permanently require canes or walkers to move around their house or outdoors. Wrist fractures of the distal radius are very common. In fact, the radius is the most commonly broken bone in the arm." Many fractures are caused by a loss of balance and an inability to recover from a fall. When we have balance, we have a greater likelihood of avoiding falls that cause fractures and trips that can send us straight to the hospital.

Endurance

Getting winded when going up stairs or running after a child is a sign of diminished heart and/or lung function. If you want to keep your heart pumping without pain and breathe freely and easily, to be able to deal with challenging situations, some form of aerobic activity is essential.

Strength

Notice how some older people have difficulty getting up out of a chair. They can't open childproof caps or jars, and they need the assistance of a cane or walker to get around. This is often due to loss of muscle mass and strength, and the only way to build or to maintain muscle is to use it. "Use it or lose it," as the saying goes. Losing it can ultimately lead to a loss of mobility and dependence on assistance from others or devices.

and

Flexibility

Lack of flexibility is a common cause of low back pain, as well as muscle aches and pains and tendon tears and ruptures. Tight muscles don't allow for blood flow and nutrients to get into the muscles or waste products, such as lactic acid, to leave the muscles. This buildup of lactic acid, which is toxic waste, causes pain, and the tightness causes imbalances and tension on the tendons. Tendons get inflamed and can tear or rupture. They take a long time to heal, and pain can be chronic. Stretching allows for increased blood flow to the area to feed the muscle and to remove waste products. It also helps you remain balanced and relieve tightness to allow for proper form when doing any other activities. All of this contributes to overall well-being and the ability to move easily and effortlessly, free from tightness, and imbalance.

Exercise Routine

Exercise can be a dirty word to some, conjuring up images of sweat, a pounding heart, and breathlessness. To some, exercise can be exhilarating and reduce stress. If you are someone who hates to exercise, you can choose to change your focus and opinions. How about calling it an activity and doing an activity that brings you pleasure?

Why Bother?

Exercise has proven benefits for everything from lowering blood pressure, weight, and cholesterol to improving mental health and kidney function and even decreasing the risk of cancer and Alzheimer's. Studies show that more physical activity was associated with a lower risk of colorectal cancer and overall mortality. Being physically fit, not smoking, and maintaining a normal waist girth are associated with lower risk of CHD (coronary heart disease) events, CVD (cardiovascular disease), and death of any cause in men. Higher levels of physical activity are associated with a lower risk of decline in kidney function. Mediterranean-type diet adherence and higher physical activity were independently associated with reduced risk for Alzheimer's disease. Aerobic and resistance exercise also results in significant, acute increases in growth hormone (GH) secretion. It is beneficial to know what type of exercise and how much exercise are enough to address your specific issues.

How to Develop Your Routine

You have the why, now let's look at the what, how much, and how often. I prescribe exercise based on many factors. One of those factors is focusing on your weak points. I would have Martha, for example, continue her walking since she enjoys it and would ask her to add some handgrip and forearm strengthening exercises, as well as something to help her with balance. For Jim, I would recommend more stretching, and adding some aerobic activity to his routine. Both would also benefit from supplements to decrease inflammation and enhance energy and tissue repair and regeneration.

Several great references for beginning or increasing your exercise routine can be found in the References. Among them is the American College of Sports Medicine, which has brochures and information on exercise guidelines, pedometers, heart rate monitors, weights, trainers, equipment, and more.

How Much? How Often?

The most important thing is to start where you are. A big mistake that people who are motivated to get started make is to do too much, too soon. This can lead to excessive soreness or injury, cause a setback, or be de-motivating. The benefit of doing baseline testing is to discover your limits and work below them. If you are not very conditioned, have injuries or weaknesses, or have musculoskeletal, heart, or lung disease, start very low and very slow to condition yourself. This is a way to safely test your limits. Always get advice from your doctor to guide you as to what is safe. Working with a trainer can be beneficial. A trainer can teach you proper form, help pace and motivate you, and change your routines to avoid boredom.

If you don't exercise regularly, you would be considered de-conditioned, and if you exercise fairly regularly, you would be considered conditioned. To avoid injury or post-exercise pain, start slowly and work up gradually. Here are some guidelines regarding how much exercise to do if you had fitness testing. If you have not had testing, do what you know you can do and follow the guidelines below.

- **De-conditioned**

  Do half of what your limit is. If you are not sore, keep adding 10% every week or two; if you are sore, cut back by 10%.

- **Conditioned**

  If you are conditioned, start with 65% of your limit and then increase by 10% every few weeks until you reach 85%. You can do more challenging aerobic routines such as interval training, which boosts growth hormone and builds cardiopulmonary function. When weight training, use the guide of 65% of your maximum limit. That will get the muscle to fatigue and work your way up slowly to 85%.

Balance

While there are no set rules for frequency and intensity, you can work up slowly and build up gradually by incorporating balance into daily exercise or everyday routines. Doing something requiring balance on a daily basis will build the muscles that support balance as well as train your nervous system to respond and recover. Here are some examples:

- Try standing on one foot while doing slow, controlled activities or while standing in line.

- Walk mindfully on uneven surfaces to build ankle strength.

- Stand on a Bosu ball and do your arm exercises with light weights, while balancing. Do them slowly and carefully.

- Step it up by balancing on one leg while standing on a Bosu ball.

- Use a balance ball to do sit-ups, push-ups, leg curls, or other moves.

- Sit on a balance ball while using light arm weights, or just sit and balance.

There are balance-related resources included in the References.

Endurance

Aerobic activity builds endurance and works your heart, lungs, and muscles. It brings circulation to your organs, tissues, and cells. Choose from a variety of activities to keep you motivated. For aerobic activity we look at being **FIT:**

Frequency

- The minimum amount of aerobic activity is five days per week.

- Moderately intense aerobic exercise 30 minutes a day, five days a week OR vigorously intense aerobic exercise 20 minutes a day, three days a week is the recommended frequency.

- If you are working at high intensity and duration, take a day off.

Intensity

- Calculate your maximum heart rate (220 minus your age) and exercise to a rate of 65 to 85% of maximum heart rate ((220 – age) x 0.65) to ((220 – age) x 0.85). I will show you how to calculate this using examples later in the text. Check your pulse or use a heart rate monitor.

- Sing-Talk Test: If you can sing while exercising, you are not working out hard enough. You should be able to talk without gasping for air. If you are gasping for air, you are working too hard and need to slow down. You can gauge the intensity of your workout by the following:

   o Mild: can talk with a slight increase in breathing

   o Moderate: can talk but need some deep breaths

   o Intense: cannot hold a conversation but not gasping for air, good for interval training. (Note: Do not do interval training until you are conditioned.)

Time

- For general health benefits: 30 minutes
- To avoid weight gain: 30–50 minutes
- For weight loss: 45–84 minutes
- To prevent weight regain after loss: 40–60 minutes

Know Your Numbers

Calculate your maximum heart rate (maximum heart rate = 220 minus your age)

Record your numbers in Appendix VI.

If you are age 50, your maximum heart rate would be 170 (220 – 50 = 170). You then calculate 65% and 85% of your maximum heart rate:

$$170 \times 0.65 = 110$$
$$170 \times 0.85 = 144$$

Your workout should be vigorous enough to get your heart rate up to 110, and you can do intervals that take you up to 144.

If you want to be more technical, there are adjustments for male and female for the maximum heart rate, but for the sake of simplicity, this works quite well.

Walking is the easiest way to get aerobic activity. Here are some tips:

- Use a pedometer and count your daily steps.
- Add 500 steps every two weeks.
- Work your way up to 10,000 steps per day.

For fun and motivation, join a walking club, an online community, or a fundraising event.

You can also perform other aerobic activities, such as:

- Elliptical
- Running
- Cycling
- Rowing
- Cross-Country Skiing
- Swimming

Schedule it, or Squeeze it In

It may take some trial and error to determine where to start. A safe way is to do what you know you can comfortably and add 10% every two weeks. Set aside time to do aerobic activity. Try different things and different times to determine what you like, and then make a plan and stick to it.

Take a class. You don't necessarily have to join a gym. Many free-standing facilities offer classes or daily access, as do some hotels. Some hospital centers now offer classes for as little as $5 per class.

Even if you travel or are stuck in meetings all day, you can squeeze in some steps by parking far from the entrance of where you are going. Take the long walk to the bathroom. Walk and talk instead of sitting in the meeting room. Find a class or a gym where you are traveling.

Strength

Strength and tone are different. As we age, we lose muscle mass and our strength decreases. Our body composition changes. We can be the same weight, but our ratio of fat to muscle changes, and we have a greater percentage of body fat compared to muscle. Strength is necessary for mobility and for tasks of daily living. To build strength, working a muscle to fatigue will build muscle mass, and that is working at 65% of your maximum.

Know Your Numbers

To gauge your strength, exercises must be performed with proper form. It's best to have a fitness trainer or trained healthcare professional, who can use instruments to measure your strength and compare you to others in your age group, test you. If you are less than average for your age, this is an area to focus on. A professional can also test more muscle groups and can look at your form. I find people who do more repetitions with poor form, are more likely to get injured and have a false sense of what they can do. If you want to try this yourself, have someone spot you, watch your form, and count; this is the next best thing.

- "1 Rep Max" is the maximum weight you can lift one time. It should be determined by a professional. If your goal is to build strength, start with 60–65% of your 1 Rep Max.

- If a professional does not test you, choose a weight that you think you can lift a few times. Perform the repetitions. If you can do three to five sets of eight to twelve repetitions before you get fatigued, this is the right weight for you.

- If you develop pain, here are some guidelines to gauge how much to do:

  o Pain after activity: decrease weight and repetitions by 25%

  o Pain during activity that does not restrict performance: decrease weight and repetitions by 50%

  o Pain during activity: stop and seek professional guidance and support

- To manage pain or stiffness:

  o Eat an anti-inflammatory diet and supplements.

(Refer to Chapter 2 and Chapter 3.)

o   Ice massage after activity.

o   Stretch.

o   Massage.

o   Drink plenty of water.

Frequency

- Do the exercises two to three days per week.

- Do eight to ten strength-training exercises: ten to fifteen repetitions of each exercise.

- Always take at least of day of rest after a weight workout.

- Muscles need time to recuperate. Near-daily training of the same muscles impairs muscle recuperation and slows progress.

Intensity

- Novice or Preparation phase: Use a weight (50–80% of your 1 Rep Max) so you can perform three to five sets of eight to twelve repetitions before the muscle gets fatigued.

- Intermediate phase: Use a heavier weight (80–90% of your 1 Rep Max) so you can perform three to five sets of one to six repetitions before the muscle gets tired.

- Vary the intensity and do recreational activities that allow you to use your muscles differently.

-

Time

- Rest three minutes between sets.

- Single-set programs: One type of exercise per muscle group is adequate.

- Multiple-set programs: Produce a greater benefit to optimize strength.

Exercises

- Squats
- Lunges
- Chest Press
- Shoulder Press
- Butterfly
- Dumbbell Fly

- Biceps Curl
- Triceps Extension
- One-Arm Row
- Lateral Raise
- Leg Press
- Leg Extension

I could write a full book on just exercise. What I am giving you here are some basic principles and guidelines. There are some great books on different types of exercise routines and websites with pictures and videos.

Flexibility

Lack of flexibility can cause pain, tightness, muscle imbalance, and poor circulation, and can make you prone to injuries and tears. My yoga class had many men in it sent by their doctors because of back pain. Stretching allows joints to move freely through full range of motion, and can correct the tightness and imbalances that put stress and strain on your joints. Just look at the soles of your shoes. We are not perfectly symmetrical. Our joints can wear unevenly if we are tighter on one side versus another, or tighter in the muscles that flex versus extend. Sitting at a computer and using a mouse is another example of how using our fingers in a flexed position all day, and cocking our wrist can cause pain in our elbows. The inflammation from repetitive use can cause swelling and nerve entrapment such as carpal tunnel syndrome.

Frequency

- After every workout, a warm muscle will stretch like taffy.
- Never stretch a cold muscle. Like taffy, it can break/tear.
- Stretch all muscle groups daily.

Intensity

- Slow and steady stretching to a point of mild discomfort
- No jerking movement

Time

- Hold stretches for twenty to thirty seconds.
- Do each stretch three to four times.

Stretches

- Inner thigh
- Low back
- Hip
- Back
- Hip Rotator
- Hamstring

- Quadricep
- Calf and Hamstring
- Achilles
- Forearm
- Shoulder
- Tendon and Calf Stretch

There are many books and websites for stretching. About.com is a good resource for descriptions of stretching exercises for various muscles. (See the References for other resources.)

Exercise Guidelines

1. Create a clear and compelling vision of who you want to be, why you want to do this, and what it will look like to maintain motivation and help you get beyond obstacles.

2. If you have any chronic medical conditions, are over the age of 50, or have not been exercising regularly, get medical clearance before starting a program. Many of the activities can be adapted for your condition, so seek expert advice.

3. Do what makes SENSE (Start Exercise Nice and Slow...Every time). Include a warm-up period along with the conditioning phase, stretching, and cool-down activities. If you stopped your exercise routine for an extended time, it's important to re-start slowly and not expect to pick up where you left off.

4. Do what you enjoy since you are most likely to stick to it.

5. Add activities that strengthen your weaknesses to avoid injury.

6. BE SaFE: Balance, Endurance (aerobics), Strength (resistance training), and Flexibility (stretching). Do something in every category and within your means, to have balanced overall fitness. Cross-train by doing different activities and changing your pattern to work different muscles and to avoid repetitive strain.

7. Be FIT. When you increase frequency (F) of exercise, cut down on the intensity (I) or the time (T) spent exercising. Alternatively, when your intensity (I) is low, you may need to exercise for a longer duration (T) to reach your goals.

8. Warm up, cool down, and stretch.

9. Drink plenty of water and avoid sugary sports drinks unless you are training for long periods of time.

10. Set goals and plan to stick to them. Make small goals that lead to larger goals or the process can seem daunting.

11. Start slowly and build up, gradually increasing duration or weight by no more than 10% at a time.

12. Listen to your body and stop if anything hurts. Get a few sessions with a trainer to assure proper form and to avoid injury, especially when lifting heavy weights. Seek professional advice when doing anything strenuous, repetitive, or out of your comfort zone.

13. Track your progress.

14. When you run up against obstacles, something is better than nothing. Just do something even if it's a stretch or another walk to the water cooler.

15. Try to be consistent and set up specific times, scheduled and on your calendar, to get some activity.

16. Congratulate yourself when you reach a milestone, celebrate success, and reward yourself with a massage, a movie, new clothing, or something that enhances your health.

Success Stories

Let's look at how exercise affected Martha and Jim.

Martha started a supplement program of Vitamin D and calcium, a good multivitamin, and fish oil. She added weight training and abdominal strengthening to her routine. Her cholesterol came down, and her bone density improved.

Jim had to back off on his upper-body training for a few weeks. He started supplements with high dose fish oil and bromelain to decrease inflammation, and he added a high-quality protein drink, high dose B vitamins, and antioxidants to aid in healing and energy production. He also began a stretching program and added aerobic activities. His rotator cuff tear was small enough that he did not need surgery. The elbow tendonitis resolved with stretching and supplements. He can still do strength training, and has a more balanced routine and better overall health.

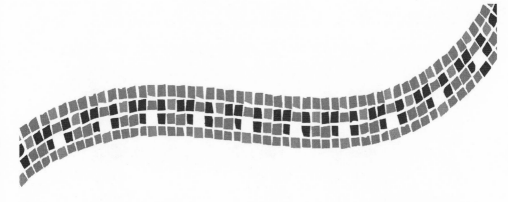

Chapter 5
Hormone Harmony

Can You Relate?

D o you eat right and exercise, yet still have some love handles? Are you tired and irritable, and can't sleep anymore? Are these symptoms interfering with your relationships, marriage, or job performance? Do you not feel like yourself anymore? Do you no longer have that ambition or competitive edge? Are you putting on weight and don't have a libido? Do you have hot flashes and night sweats? Are you itchy or bitchy, and don't even want to try sex because you are so dry?

Hormone imbalances or deficiencies may be the culprit.

Elizabeth, a 38-year-old, has a good life, wonderful children, and a supportive husband. She works part-time from home because she wants to, not because she has to. However, at a certain time of the month she becomes angry and irritable, and she doesn't sleep. She snaps at her husband and children. She doesn't know what comes over her and feels out of control. She is afraid her husband will leave her if this continues.

Matthew, a 45-year-old, is the CEO of a mid-sized company. He was always athletic and on the top of his game. He is newly married to a young wife and has it all: the money, car, family, a great job with power and position.

Yet he doesn't feel right. He was told his health is good. He had a full evaluation at a high-priced executive health clinic, yet no one could get to the bottom of his feelings of listlessness, his dissatisfaction with himself, and the decline of his athletic abilities, as well as his thickening waistline. His libido and sex life were also less than satisfactory, and this was causing him some anxiety. He was told it was his age.

Jeanine, a 58-year-old executive, is beside herself. She has hot flashes during meetings, wakes up at night drenched in sweat, and can't go back to sleep. Her memory is poor, and she can't remember names. Her skin is dry and lifeless, and vaginal dryness makes sex painful, so she avoids it. She gained ten pounds all around her midsection and is getting depressed because she feels her life and health are deteriorating.

Many of the symptoms described can be related to hormones that are too high, too low, or out of balance. Nothing stirs more controversy in the medical and lay community than the topic of hormones. It conjures up images of sports figures testifying before Congress, pumped-up, muscle-bound people, or thoughts of hormones being bad or wrong. Hormones are a necessary part of our very existence. Here's the definition of hormone: a chemical substance produced in the body that controls and regulates the activity of certain cells or organs. We need hormones to regulate cell activity, communicate with our DNA to regenerate or repair damaged cell and tissues, communicate with our immune systems to fight infections, and turn protein production and cell division or cell death on or off. Each hormone has its own cycle and rhythm, and hormones perform many functions. Since this is just an overview, I will only highlight some hormones that you can modulate with lifestyle and some of their major functions.

Here's a list of some hormones that are necessary to function optimally:

- Cortisol
- DHEA
- Estrogen
- Growth Hormone

- Insulin
- Pregnenolone
- Progesterone

- Testosterone
- Thyroid
- Vitamin D

As we age, cortisol and insulin increase, and all of the rest listed above decrease. Like anything in nature, we are born to reproduce and then die. This cascade of hormone depletion signals the body that we have fulfilled our purpose to reproduce and that it's time for the next generation to take over. However, we are now living way beyond our reproductive years, and these hormone deficiencies or imbalances can have some serious health effects.

Each hormone has a counter hormone. Some hormones build tissues, such as DHEA and testosterone, and others break them down, like cortisol. Glucagon raises blood sugar, and insulin lowers it. Everything must be in balance for us to have good health.

It is standard care to replace some hormones that are low, such as insulin, thyroid, and Vitamin D. In fact, it would be malpractice not to. However, there are no such generally accepted guidelines and practices regarding replacing low levels of some of the other hormones, despite evidence that they could be beneficial. There may be risks to replacing any hormone if too much is given, and there are also risks of allowing levels to drop too low. I encourage readers, as I do my patients, to educate themselves and talk to a health care professional with experience monitoring hormone replacement.

Estrogen and Progesterone

Estrogen signals the uterine lining to grow. On a monthly basis, most women get a progesterone surge. This stabilizes uterine lining growth to prepare the uterus for pregnancy. If an egg does not get fertilized and implanted, both drop, and menses occur. If estrogen, a stimulating hormone, is not balanced with progesterone, a calming hormone, it can lead to fibroids, fibrocystic breasts, and PMS-like symptoms, as well as irritability and insomnia, among other things. This is very common in the early teenage years when hormone cycles are being activated, as well as in the peri-menopausal phase, when ovulation is sporadic, progesterone is not being produced on a regular basis, and estrogen is.

Creating a better balance by lowering estrogen can alleviate symptoms of peri-menopause. If you choose not to replace progesterone, try soluble fiber, which can bind excess estrogen and eliminate it from your body. Many of my patients do very well for some time with dietary changes alone.

During menopause, in most women, estrogen and progesterone drop, and some women get the "Seven Dwarfs of Menopause," made popular by Suzanne Somers: itchy, bitchy, sweaty, bloaty, sleepy, forgetful, and psycho. Estrogen acts on the pituitary to control body temperature, keeps skin soft and supple, enhances memory, prevents bone loss, and more. Progesterone acts as a diuretic and promotes restful sleep, as well as modulates mood swings.

Herbs such as black cohosh, chasteberry, and rhapontic rhubarb are the most efficacious herbs studied that can relieve some symptoms of peri-menopause or menopause, especially hot flashes. These can be found as part of a mixed formula or as individual supplements taken as directed by the manufacturer. There are great variations in herbal extracts, and I recommend you buy them from a reputable company.

Testosterone

When testosterone drops in men, they lose muscle and bone mass. They complain of tiredness, lack of energy, reduced strength, frailty, loss of libido, decreased sexual performance, depression, and mood change. Women have some testosterone, too. It strengthens bones, stabilizes mood, and gives self-confidence.

Testosterone can be made more bioavailable with herbs. In men, weight-lifting can also elevate testosterone.

There is a lot of controversy regarding hormone replacement therapy, and whether or not you choose to replenish your hormones is a personal choice. The American Society of Andrology's position is that "testosterone replacement therapy in aging men is indicated when both clinical symptoms and signs suggestive of androgen deficiency and decreased testosterone levels are present." The American College of Obstetrics and Gynecology's position on hormone replacement therapy in symptomatic women is as follows: "…take the smallest dose of hormone therapy that works for you, for the shortest amount of time."

Control Cortisol and Insulin to Age Less

A whole series of textbooks could be devoted to this topic alone, and, since this is a self-help guide, we will focus on two major hormones that you can modulate with diet, exercise, and supplements: cortisol and insulin. These hormones are linked to many of the chronic degenerative diseases of aging and are interrelated. Both respond to blood sugar levels. Cortisol increases when blood sugar is low and will elevate it, and insulin is produced when blood sugar is high and will lower it. The fluctuation between the two creates a hormone roller coaster that wreaks havoc on your health.

Cortisol

The most common things I see in my practice are stress-related signs and symptoms, such as fluctuating energy levels, loss of muscle mass, and fat around the middle.

One of the culprits is cortisol. Cortisol is released in response to stress. The stress can be physical (too hot, too cold, pain, etc.) or mental (worry, financial woes, relationship issues, and even happy occasions like a promotion or excitement from an adrenaline rush). Cortisol is an essential hormone that regulates your immune system, prepares you for a state of emergency, and puts you on high alert. It is essential for you to respond to a threat — the "fight or flight" response. Most stress no longer requires a physical fight or flight. However, we are programmed to release this hormone anyway. A short-term release of this hormone is necessary, but when you are subject to chronic, ongoing stress, the ongoing release of this hormone has negative effects.

Excess cortisol increases the following:

- Storage of fat
- Blood sugar
- Blood pressure
- Cholesterol

- Triglycerides
- Insulin
- Cravings
- Binge eating

Excess cortisol decreases the following:

- Muscle and bone mass
- Mental clarity
- Sensitivity to insulin
- Sleep
- Memory

Excess cortisol can worsen the following conditions:

- Menopause
- Sleep disturbances
- Andropause
- Aging
- Premenstrual syndrome (PMS)
- Worry
- Irritable bowel
- And more.
- Confusion

Too little would put you in a state of collapse. Your blood pressure and blood sugar would drop, your immune system can be over-stimulated, and allergies get worse, fatigue sets in, your thyroid won't function well, wounds don't heal, menopausal and perimenopausal symptoms worsen, and a sense of fatigue, overwhelm, and lack of motivation ensues.

The main things that stimulate cortisol release are stress and worry, fluctuations in blood sugar, and stimulants. A diet high in sugar, alcohol, refined carbohydrates, and white, starchy foods will increase insulin. However, since blood sugar rises fast when eating highly refined or processed foods and insulin production lags behind, insulin reaches its peak when your blood sugar levels are low and drives the level further down. This causes low blood sugar or hypoglycemia. This is perceived as a physical stress by the body and stimulates the release of cortisol. The dip in blood sugar is usually felt as fatigue, headache, lightheadedness, and a craving for sugar or refined carbohydrates, leading to cravings and binge eating. This cyclical roller-coaster ride will continue until you intervene by stopping the wild swings in blood sugar. The guidance in Chapter 2 outlines not only what, but also how, you eat controls this cortisol/blood sugar/insulin response.

Going too long without eating does the same thing. Blood sugar levels drop, you become hypoglycemic, you eat a large meal, insulin production lags behind and reaches its peak when blood sugar has dropped, causing a further drop, and the cycle continues.

This is the reason why vegetables and complex carbohydrates are so important. They take time to digest, and they release glucose slowly, decrease the insulin response, modulate mood and appetite, and provide more nutrients needed to regenerate and repair tissues and replenish cortisol.

It takes a lot of energy to go through these cycles and swings, and to make cortisol. Your body uses more B vitamins, Vitamin C, and magnesium, and we have already seen that much of the population is deficient in some of these. Having adequate nutrition is essential to managing stress. Eating small, frequent meals of nutrient-dense, anti-inflammatory foods high in antioxidants is an essential component of hormone management as well as stress management.

Tips to manage cortisol:

- Practice stress-management techniques.

- Eat small, frequent meals.

- Limit sugar, alcohol, caffeine, refined carbohydrates, and white foods such as white bread, pasta, rice, and potatoes.

- Supplement with a B50 complex, at least 1,000–3,000 mg of Vitamin C, and 200–600 mg of magnesium.

- Use adaptogenic herb preparations such as ashwaganda, rhodeola, and/or ginseng.

- Use calming herbs such as valerian, lemon balm, chamomile, hops, and/or passion flower.

- Phosphatidyl serine (300 mg per day) can protect your hypothalamus from the damaging effects of high levels of cortisol and preserve memory.

- L theanine (100 mg three times a day) can keep you calm yet alert.

Insulin

Insulin is the hormone that regulates blood sugar. It does this by signaling the liver to stop making glucose (a form of sugar) and allows glucose (sugar) to enter your cells. Glucose enters your cells so it can be used as a fuel source or stored in your muscles as glycogen, a reservoir of energy, for when you need it. If the glycogen storage areas are full, it stores the excess as fat, usually around your midsection.

Remember that insulin requires receptors on cell surfaces, which act like a doorman with a lock and key to allow entrance of glucose into a cell. Without insulin and a receptor, glucose can't get into your cells, and the cells without a source of fuel for energy die. When receptors get saturated or full, blocked, or decrease in numbers, excess glucose circulates in your body and can bind to protein, causing damage. This damage is called glycation and is the same as the process of caramelization of a sugar-coated ham. It forms a nice crust. Diabetics have this going on most of the time at an accelerated rate, and all of these are complications of diabetes. However, it can occur in low levels in non-diabetics and contributes to many of the aforementioned chronic degenerative diseases of aging.

Your body makes insulin in response to glucose. The higher the level, the more insulin is made. However, this overwhelms the receptors and you get insulin resistance. A simple analogy to describe what happens when you get insulin resistance is that the excess glucose overwhelms the receptors and stops working. (The lock jams, and the doorman gets overwhelmed and can't handle the load.)

Insulin also takes excess glucose and stores it as fat in your midsection as triglycerides. High fasting insulin does not allow active muscle cells to take up glucose as easily as they should. In that situation, the blood insulin levels are chronically high, which inhibits our fat cells from giving up their energy stores to let us lose weight. This is a sign of Syndrome X, otherwise known as metabolic syndrome.

Insulin resistance is associated with obesity, high blood pressure, abnormal triglycerides, glucose intolerance, and type 2 diabetes mellitus. Many women with polycystic ovaries have this, as well as women who have gestational diabetes in pregnancy. Up to 50% of patients with hypertension are estimated to have insulin resistance. Metabolic syndrome is a group of risk factors that increases your risk of heart disease, stroke, and diabetes. A factor in developing metabolic syndrome, which is now epidemic, is insulin resistance. This is why measuring your blood pressure, fasting blood sugar, waist and hip sizes, and blood lipids (cholesterol, triglycerides, HDL, and LDL) is important. Measuring fasting insulin can also be revealing. If it's high when you haven't had any glucose or food to stimulate its production, you have insulin resistance and are well on your way to developing diabetes, heart and blood vessel disease, and all of their complications.

According to the American Heart Association and the National Heart, Lung, and Blood Institute, metabolic syndrome is present if you have three or more of the following signs:

- Blood pressure equal to or higher than 130/85 mmHg
- Fasting blood sugar (glucose) equal to or higher than 100 mg/dL
- Large waist circumference (length around the waist):
  o Men: 40 inches or more
  o Women: 35 inches or more
- Low HDL cholesterol:
  o Men: under 40 mg/dL
  o Women: under 50 mg/dL
- Triglycerides equal to or higher than 150 mg/dL

Insulin receptor sensitivity can be enhanced by:

- Weight loss if you are overweight
- Eating small, frequent meals to maintain a level blood glucose
- A diet low in sugar, alcohol, refined carbohydrates, and white foods such as white bread, pasta, rice, potato, corn, and starchy vegetables
- Exercising to increase insulin receptor sensitivity and to help you lose weight
- Chromium
- Cinnamon
- Fish oil
- Alpha lipoic acid

Success Stories

Let's look at how modulating hormones through diet and supplementation affected Elizabeth, Matthew, and Jeanine.

Elizabeth had her hormones tested. She had high levels of estrogen and little to no progesterone due to lack of ovulation. Testosterone levels were also low. Her cortisol levels were high, and all other hormones were normal. She was told to eliminate processed foods and cut down on sugar, refined carbohydrates, caffeine, and alcohol, and was prescribed high dose pharmaceutical-grade B 50 complex, Vitamin C, magnesium, fish oil, phosphatidylserine, L theanine, and soluble fiber. She was also prescribed oral bioidentical progesterone and bioidentical testosterone cream. She called me a week after her next period started so excited because she slept, and felt calm and at peace. Her husband noticed the difference and was very appreciative. She felt like herself again and in better control of her life and emotions.

Matthew had his hormones evaluated and was found to be low on testosterone. He was prescribed a testosterone cream with chrysin to help avoid hair loss. He was asked to exercise with weights, as well as do some cardiovascular interval training. His cortisol levels were low, and he was told to eliminate processed foods and cut down on sugar, refined carbohydrates, caffeine, and alcohol. He was prescribed high dose pharmaceutical-grade B 50 complex, Vitamin C, magnesium, fish oil, and adaptogenic herbs. Several months later he returned with a smile on his face. He lost fifteen pounds, had energy and vitality, and got his confidence back. His relationship with his wife improved, and he felt at the top of his game at work.

Jeanine had low levels of estrogen, progesterone, and cortisol and DHEA. She was told to eliminate processed foods and cut down on sugar, refined carbohydrates, caffeine, and alcohol, and she was prescribed high dose pharmaceutical-grade B 50 complex, Vitamin C, magnesium, fish oil, and adaptogenic herbs. She was prescribed bioidentical estrogen and progesterone, and was given DHEA. She returned in a few months and said her symptoms had improved. She still has night sweats and hot flashes, but they are much less frequent, and she sleeps much better. Her energy levels are still low. Repeat testing showed all her levels were improved but still low. Her estrogen and progesterone were increased, and she was told to rest when she needed to and not push herself, as well as to practice stress-management techniques. Several months later she returned with a newfound energy and enthusiasm. She no longer had hot flashes or night sweats. Her sleep was sound, and her memory improved. She said she felt the best she had in years.

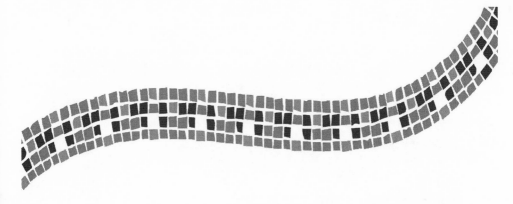

Chapter 6
Stress Less, Age Less

Can You Relate?

Do you feel tense, irritable, or overwhelmed? Do you have headaches, insomnia, muscles tightness, fatigue, mental fog, or poor memory?

> Rita, a 49-year-old, complained of anxiety. She was feeling irritable and overwhelmed, as well as fatigued. She was not her usual energetic self, and she thought she was approaching menopause since everything else in her life was stable.
>
> Tony, a 50-year-old, experienced insomnia and short bouts of fatigue. He had back pain, and felt stiff and sore. He had a high-powered job, and he loved the excitement and challenge.

Many of the symptoms described here could be due to stress; however, it is important to have an evaluation by your doctor to be sure you don't have an underlying medical condition. The stress response occurs when you perceive a threat. Your brain releases signals that increase the output of neurotransmitters (signals to your nervous system) and hormones. These tell your body to make adrenaline and cortisol to raise your blood pressure and blood sugar, to increase your heart rate, and to divert energy to your muscles and away from your gastrointestinal and immune systems. It decreases your desire to reproduce and grow since all energy is diverted to systems that allow you to flee. You are in high-alert mode.

The stress response is vital to our survival. Our heart pounds; blood rushes to our muscles and away from our immune, digestive, and other systems; our pupils dilate so we can see our predator; and adrenaline and cortisol pump to increase glucose, blood pressure, heart rate, and sweat. All are adaptive responses to the fight or flight syndrome. However, when your computer malfunctions, your children are misbehaving, your boss or customers are irate and applying pressure or unrealistic expectations, you still respond the same — even though it does no good, and actually hurts you in the long run!

Stress can have a negative influence on many conditions. Here's a small sample:

- Depression
- Diabetes
- Hair loss
- Heart disease
- Hyperthyroidism
- Obesity
- Obsessive-compulsive disorder
- Anxiety disorder
- Sexual dysfunction
- Tooth and gum disease
- Ulcers
- Cancer

If you can't change a situation, change your reaction to it. This is easier said than done because we are hard-wired to respond to fight or flee, and our culture does not train us in healthy adaptive responses.

We can learn a lot from Eastern cultures about being present, accepting, and forgiving, as well as adopting an attitude of gratitude. Yogi and Zen masters teach these concepts as a form of spiritual enlightenment. They are simple and elegant, yet at times they can be difficult to master.

Stress can age us prematurely, and managing the stress response is vital to our health. Yet, there is more than just the physical dynamics to master and practicing the stress-reduction tips at the end of this chapter. There are attitudinal dynamics that play a role in how we age, experience joy, and navigate life with grace and ease. Aging well can be done.

George Vaillant, MD, a respected professor of psychiatry at Harvard Medical School, conducted a study. The Harvard Study of Adult Development was the longest, most comprehensive examination of aging ever conducted. Since the 1930s, researchers have studied more than 800 men and women, following them from adolescence into old age, and seeking clues to the behaviors that translate into happy and healthy longevity. John Mitchell, MD, wrote: "Dr. Vaillant suggests that successful aging means giving to others joyously whenever one is able; receiving from others, gratefully, whenever one needs it; and being capable of personal development in between."

There is personal power in adapting an attitude of gratitude, since we send out vibes to attract to us what we put out. In the people who aged well, he found that healthy individuals adopted attitudes of gratitude, forgiveness, and joy. They accepted their fate in a genuine way, and had a future orientation, loving relationships, and a strong social network. He acknowledged that people can change. You, by picking up this book, can be one of these people. What kind of attitude will you adopt?

Dan Buettner, author of *The Blue Zones: Lessons for Living Longer,* hired longevity researchers to identify pockets in places around the world where people are living longer with great health. In these Blue Zones, they found people who reach age 100 at rates ten times greater than in the United States. The people in the Blue Zones had a fraction of the rate of heart disease and cancer that we do, and they live up to ten years longer with strength, vigor, and vitality.

They had several things in common, such as:

- A strong commitment to family and social ties
- A Mediterranean diet, mostly plant-based with lots of legumes
- Exercise as a daily part of life, well into their golden years
- A sense of purpose
- Strong social networks and community networks
- Not smoking

If you think this can only happen in places like Sardinia, Italy;

Nacoya Peninsula, Costa Rica; and Icaria, Greece, and that it's not possible in a modern society, think again: Loma Linda, California was also a Blue Zone.

It's possible to live longer and healthier, and to manage stress. Stress will happen. If we happen to find ourselves in stressful situations, here are some tips to diffuse and/or relieve stress.

Breathing

Taking deep, slow, mindful breaths is an ancient practice that has many benefits. It is one of my very favorite forms of stress relief. Breathing exercises are excellent, are free, and can be done anytime and anywhere. They work well by increasing your vagal tone (the nerve system that slows heart rate, lowers blood pressure, slows pulse rate, and calms your system down). Taking deep, slow breaths breaks the cycle of the outpouring of sympathetic tone (adrenaline causes the racing heart, sweaty palms, and elevation of blood pressure) and cortisol. Deep, controlled breathing is calming. If you can catch yourself and control your breath when you're in the middle of a very stressful situation, you can stop the stress reaction dead in its tracks. Here's how:

- Sit or stand in a relaxed position.
- Slowly inhale through your nose, counting to five in your head.
- Let the air out from your mouth, counting to eight in your head as it leaves your lungs.
- Repeat several times. That's it!

Tips:

- As you breathe, let your abdomen expand outward. This is a more relaxed and natural way to breathe, and helps your lungs fill themselves more fully with fresh air, releasing more carbon dioxide waste.
- You can do this just a few times to release tension, or for several minutes as a form of meditation.
- If you like, you can make your throat a little tighter as you

exhale so the air comes out like a whisper. This type of breathing is used in some forms of yoga and can add additional tension relief.

Progressive Muscle Relaxation

Tensing and relaxing muscles is a very basic stress reliever. It's simple and easy to learn, and with practice you can reduce or eliminate the tension in your entire body in a matter of seconds. Mindfully tense each muscle as tight as you can, hold for a few seconds and relax so you can feel the difference. Start with your feet and work your way up your body, keeping any part that was tensed and relaxed in a relaxed state. Allow the state of relaxation to move up your body. Remain in this relaxed state for at least five minutes.

Meditation

Meditation is one of the most effective and widely practiced stress relievers around. It takes regular practice and can feel awkward at times, but there are so many benefits. It increases vagal tone, which is very calming. Meditation is an excellent form of stress relief, and can even help prevent future stress. There are many types of meditations to try; you can meditate by sitting on the beach listening to the waves, sitting in front of a crackling fire and staring, staring at a candle flame, repeating a mantra or phrase over and over again, or walking mindfully in nature, emptying your mind of thoughts. The important part is letting your thoughts go and going back to listening to your breath, the waves, or a sound, or looking at a point of focus. Detach from your thoughts and watch them as if they were leaves on a stream floating away. You can buy guided tapes or just focus on your breath going in and going out, letting any intrusive thoughts go. The important thing is to just do it.

Exercise

Exercise relieves tension and gets blood circulating throughout your body, and it can take you out of your head. Do something you enjoy. Take a walk with a friend, try a workout video in your home, go to a class or a gym, or take a bike ride. Whatever you choose, you can experience the release of tension and the influx of endorphins that accompany exercise — and it doesn't cost a thing.

Laughter

It not only diffuses a tense situation, but laughter is often called "the best medicine." A deep belly laugh is a fun, free stress reliever. Maintaining a sense of humor in life helps you to take things less seriously; it can be a great way to relieve stress and can make life more enjoyable at the same time. It can relieve stress in those around you as well.

Music

Listening to music has many proven benefits. It's enjoyable, effortless, and readily available. Choose music to alter your mood. To calm yourself, listen to meditation, classical, or other relaxing music to soothe your body, or listen to upbeat music to create energy and lift your mood.

Saying No

Re-examining priorities and saying no can help you set boundaries and reduce stress before you experience it. This can free up your time for other activities, and relieve the stress and pressure of being overwhelmed and stressing over a lengthy to-do list.

Yoga

Yoga is one of the oldest self-improvement practices around, dating back over five thousand years! It combines the practices of several other stress-management techniques, such as breathing, meditation, imagery, and movement, giving you a lot of benefit for the amount of time and energy required. It is one of my favorites. There is a deep philosophy that can be grounding and applied to everyday encounters.

Success Stories

Let's look at how managing stress affected Rita and Tony.

Rita had her hormone levels checked, and I showed her that her cortisol level spiked high mid-day. When I asked her what happened at that time of day, she cried. Her daughter was jobless, moved back home, and was not actively looking for work. Although Rita was functioning quite well, the stress was having a physiologic affect on her and her health. Once she became aware of this, she prepared herself for confronting her daughter by seeking counseling, a way of reframing the situation, practiced saying no, and began a prayer practice. While she couldn't change the situation, she was able to change her reaction to it. She felt more at peace accepting the situation for what it is and focusing on what she could change: herself.

Tony had cortisol spikes at night just before going to bed and realized he spent time ruminating and planning, which interrupted his sleep. He was asked to write things down, not eat late, and take magnesium, calming herbs, and phosphatidly serine before bedtime. He eliminated processed foods and cut down on sugar, refined carbohydrates, caffeine, and alcohol. He was prescribed high dose pharmaceutical-grade B 50 complex, Vitamin C, and fish oil to take during the day. He also agreed to try yoga for his back pain, and he reports that his symptoms are much improved.

My parting advice:

- Love and appreciate yourself.
- Laugh often.
- Spend time in nature.
- Spend time with your family and friends.

Life is to be lived with joy, love, and laughter with family and friends, expressing ourselves fully and living healthfully to our full potential. A healthy mind and body make our trip through life that much more enjoyable.

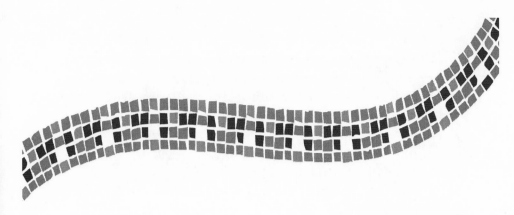

Chapter 7
Beyond the Basics

The power of the synergistic effects of diet, exercise, supplements, and hormone modulation cannot be underestimated. Many of my patients experience profound differences with these basic changes. Those who make positive changes in all of these areas have a greater impact than those who do some. Even those who take only some of the steps find improved health and well-being. Don't underestimate the impact of an optimal nutrition, supplement, and exercise program, controlling your hormone response, and handling stress better. These are foundational elements that can give you a good night's sleep, mental clarity, pain relief, increased energy, strength, endurance, balance, and flexibility; enhance your immune system; and modulate illness, making you less reliant on medication.

Yet, some people may not respond as well as others. Why? Some try some or all recommendations for a few weeks and lose motivation; others don't want to change their diet or take supplements or do any activity. And there are others who seem to be doing all of the right things and can't seem to turn things around.

Uniquely You

We are all unique, and the way we metabolize is different. Our metabolic pathways to transform food into energy and to modulate all of the complex, inter-related processes that go on in our bodies, hasn't changed much. However, our environment has. Our knowledge of how things work and the influence of genetics, environment, and lifestyle is exploding. Through science, patience, and perseverance we can unlock the secrets of your genetic and metabolic codes, and utilize environmental and lifestyle changes to work with your individual needs and metabolic and genetic profile to transform your life and health.

If the basics don't get you where you want to go, I encourage you to dig deeper and go further. Some people go to different healthcare practitioners for different things. Your plan may be piecemeal and contain conflicting advice with no communication among your various practitioners. You may be left on your own to sort things out. Other people go for a major work-up at a high-priced clinic and find out they don't have cancer or cardiovascular disease. They may get some peace of mind, but they still don't feel well and are lost to follow up. Many of my patients are on a multitude of medications and want a different approach. My approach is to look deeper at how an individual metabolizes, what the genetic and lifestyle influences are on their metabolism, understanding their risk factors and assisting them in reducing those risks, measuring deficiencies and biomarkers to get an understanding of their needs, and customizing their diet, supplements, exercise regime, and lifestyle to address their unique issues. I will give you an idea of how to evaluate some of these.

Metabolic and Disease Process

The development of disease is a process. Managing only one part of the process leaves you open to the other parts being left unattended, which can wreak havoc on your health. Everything you eat, breathe, or put on your skin gets absorbed and processed, or transformed into something else, using enzymes and nutrients. These processes transform food into energy, neutralize toxins, and remove waste. Each substance goes through several steps, and enzymes and nutrient cofactors facilitate every step in its breakdown or transformation. This is metabolism. The steps in a metabolic process are like a factory assembly line. I love the *I Love Lucy* skit where she couldn't package the candy fast enough. The line backed up, candy went all over the place, she stuffed some in her mouth, some fell on the floor, and the whole assembly line broke down. The backed-up candy at the beginning of the line and the empty boxes at the end of the line indicated something was wrong with the process.

You have heard the phrase "where there is smoke, there is fire." In medicine, the smoke, or some might call it a red flag, is a biomarker. A biomarker is something you can measure and is a component in a step of a metabolic process. When a biomarker is too high or too low, it means there is a problem with that process. It tells us where we should look or where the problems are. Knowing your biomarkers of processes that accelerate damage or aging, such as inflammation, oxidation, or glycation, can indicate the dietary, supplement, or lifestyle interventions that can bypass the block, take away the block, or give what is needed to allow the process to function optimally.

Let's use an example of an oversimplified metabolic process where:

1. **Candy** is substance A. In science we call this substrate A or biomarker A.

2. The **worker** is enzyme AB to allow the process to go from A to B. The process here is getting candy into the box. Each worker is different even though they are all doing the same job. They respond differently to the environment, which can make them work more or less efficiently.

3. The **box** is substrate B or biomarker B.

4. The motor to run the **assembly line** requires energy or power (enzymes) and many moving parts (cofactors such as vitamins or nutrients).

5. A **monkey wrench** is an expression of an outside influence that can slow or stop a process. In the medical sense it can be attributed to a toxin, trauma, infection, or other outside force that interferes with everything running smoothly.

Metabolic Pathway

In order to get from A to B, or to get candy in the box, we need all of the above. If you are not getting the desired outcome — the right amount of candy in the box, which we will use as an analogy for optimum health — we need to look at the entire process.

- **Biomarker:** The first signs of something being wrong are too much candy backing up at the beginning of the assembly line, and empty or partially filled boxes at the end. The candy backlog and empty boxes are signs or biomarkers that you can measure. A biomarker that is too high or too low means your health is not optimal.

- **Genetic single nucleotide polymorphism, or SNP:** We can test for worker variability. Say the normal variant is a worker with two arms that was trained to do the job and can work at a certain speed. If the worker only has one arm (a genetic variant) we would have to change the speed (the environment) or add another worker or make some kind of modification. Some workers work better when it's warm, and others work better when it's cold. Some have preferences that allow them to work better and faster. These preferences or genetic variations can be determined with testing for SNPs.

- **Enzymes and Nutrients, or Cofactors:** Bringing the candy to the worker at a certain speed in an organized process requires an assembly line, which requires energy or power, and mechanical parts to run. Enxymes are required to help the metabolic transformation work. Nutrients, act as cofactors and help enzymes work by catalyzing the reactions. We can look at the levels of nutrients and determine if they are at optimal levels to get the job done well.

- **Environmental factors:** A monkey wrench such as worker illness or absence can slow or stop the process. We sometimes have to look at outside influences to find out why the process is not running smoothly. It can be anything, such as stress, lack of fitness, infection, trauma, toxins, temperature, or other factors. There are many things to look at. However, if we only look at part of the process, we may miss something.

Metabolic Processes of Aging

Let's take this a step further and look at how we age. Like anything in nature, we burn, we brown, we rust, our hormones and nervous systems decline, and we succumb to illness, infection, trauma, toxins, or other outside influences. Metabolically, these processes are called inflammation, glycation, oxidation, and neuroendocrine decline. Remember that these processes were discussed in previous chapters; now we will look at them in the context of an aging metabolism and the biomarkers they produce.

- **Inflammation** is implicated, as you recall, in the development of many diseases such as Alzheimer's, autoimmune disease, cancer, and more. It can be dramatic and give a clear signal, expressing as full-blown diseases already mentioned, or it can be a low-grade, smoldering condition that is not easily detected. One of the biomarkers of inflammation is C-reactive protein, or CRP. The fatty acids in our body regulate inflammation, and they have to be in balance. A fatty acid profile and Omega 3 index can give us valuable information regarding whether we have what it takes to manage inflammation.

- **Glycation** is discussed in detail in Chapter 2; there are more details about the process of sugar binding to proteins and how the changes in structure of those proteins changes the way they function, such as clouding of the lenses in your eyes or disrupting signals in your brain or the filtering process in your kidneys. A biomarker of glycation is Hemoglobin A1C, or HbgA1C.

- **Oxidation**, or rusting, is the formation of free radicals that cause cell death and accelerate inflammation. Free radicals are the end product of many metabolic processes, such as eating, breathing, and exercising. There are many biomarkers for oxidative stress. One is 8-Hydroxy-2'-deoxyguanosine, or 8-OHdG. 8-OHdG is a product of oxidative damage by free radicals to DNA, and the 8-OHdG test tells you if you have enough antioxidants in your system. Two others are malondialdehyde and thiobarbituric acid, markers for lipid oxidation, which has been linked to genetic mutation and cancer. We can also look at pathways that involve antioxidants such as alpha lipoic acid, glutathione, and vitamins such as Vitamin A, Vitamin C, and Vitamin E. A slowdown will show up if you don't have enough of these nutrients. Having adequate antioxidant protection is important to maintain health.

- **Neuroendocrine decline** occurs when our neurotransmitters and hormones decline or become out of balance. These can be measured, balanced, and replaced. Looking at the entire process of how these are made, which is called the pathway, we can determine if there are any blocks, toxic byproducts, or deficiencies. By correcting deficiencies or giving something to speed up or slow down an enzyme, we can redirect the pathway, neutralize toxic by-products and allow the process to flow more smoothly in the direction we want. We can also apply the same principles to measuring the pathway of production of neurotransmitters made from amino acids (the breakdown products of protein). Neurotransmitters regulate cell communication, mood, and the functioning of our nervous system.

- **Environmental factors** such as stress, infection, and trauma, toxic overload, or other outside forces can affect our health and accelerate the aging process. Organic acids give us feedback about the pathways that produce energy and can give us insights into where the breakdown is occurring. An organic acid profile measures where the backup is and can give us indications if nutritional deficiencies or environmental factors come into play. We can also run other tests that look for infection, the effects of toxins, metabolic functions of our organ systems, allergies, autoimmune disease, and more.

These processes go on all over our bodies and influence many chronic degenerative diseases of aging, such as arthritis, allergy, asthma, autoimmune disease, cancer, diabetes, and more. They also contribute to the mild aches and pains, mental fog, gastric upset, and other minor maladies that interrupt our well-being.

As you can see, it's never one thing. To truly understand your unique differences, there is nothing better than a customized approach to unlock the secrets of your individual genetic variants, metabolic pathways, and physical, mental, and nutritional status. If you want to unlock your genetic and metabolic codes, have a thorough workup with an anti-aging, metabolic specialist well trained and well versed in the application and interpretation of cutting-edge, evidenced-based medicine and the synergistic power of advanced testing, optimized nutrition, supplements, hormones, exercise, stress management, attitude, and lifestyle. You deserve a customized approach to your individual needs since one size does not fit all.

Let's explore how a customized approach can transform your health, looking at some common ailments that are interrelated because they stem from the same processes listed above. Once you understand one process, the same principles apply to all, though the biomarkers and tests you do to uncover problems may differ. Let's explore the frontier of anti-aging, metabolic medicine, and epigenetics.

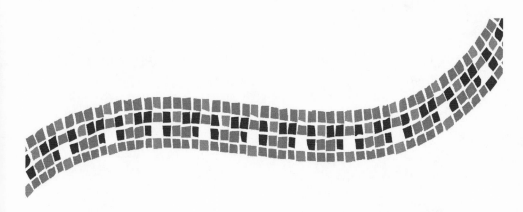

Chapter 8
Customized Care

Now that you understand what metabolism is and how looking deeper can uncover breakdowns that serve as red flags, we will look at one organ system as an example of how to apply the principles of metabolic medicine to uncover issues and customize an approach. Your heart and blood vessels, otherwise known as the cardiovascular system, are responsible for delivering vital nutrients to every cell, tissue, and organ in your body, as well as carrying waste products to the liver and kidneys for detoxification and elimination. They feed everything, including your brain, and lie at the very "heart" of health. I will use this system to illustrate how the processes we looked at are the basis of cardiovascular as well as other disease, and how we can modulate them using customized testing and individualized prescriptions of nutrition, supplements, fitness, lifestyle, and stress management.

There are many factors that put your cardiovascular system at risk, which not only affects the heart and blood vessels, but every organ in your body. Focusing on only one risk factor, such as cholesterol, is like saying a plant only needs water, without regard to sunlight and the quality of the soil. Giving a plant everything it needs to thrive will allow it to thrive and bloom. The same is true of your cardiovascular and other organ systems.

The Process of Plaque

Cardiovascular disease is disease of your heart, blood vessels, and everything they feed. The process by which disease develops is an inflammatory process. Free radicals in your body oxidize cholesterol. Then, the oxidized cholesterol attracts cells that start the inflammatory process. The oxidized cholesterol sticks to your artery walls and gets between the cells; the inflammation causes the cholesterol to harden, which is called plaque. Plaques build up and begin narrowing the artery — your source of oxygen and nutrients that keep cells alive and functioning normally. The inflammatory process causes damage to the artery walls that are plugged up by clotting factors and blood clots form over the plaque.

Go With the Flow

Your arteries are elastic and can stretch and contract to meet the demands of blood flow when you are standing, sitting, lying down, walking, running, or resting. The flow has to change according to the demand: Running will require more blood flow, oxygen, and nutrients than sitting and reading a book. When you are standing, blood could pool in your legs if the flow was not adjusted to pump more to your head. The arteries in your legs will narrow to direct more blood flow to your head so you won't faint. Thus, the elasticity of your arteries is very important to direct blood flow and control pressure. Lack of pressure can cause you to pass out or cause damage to areas where the flow is low. High pressure can put a strain on your heart and cause weakened areas of your arteries to burst. Plaques make your blood vessels rigid so they can't adjust to the changing needs, and they can also weaken the blood vessel walls, so you can see why hardening of the arteries can be a problem affecting every organ of your body.

What Is an Infarct?

That hardened plaque attracts clotting factors from your blood, and blood clots form. As this process builds, the plaque becomes unstable and breaks off. These pieces can lodge in your brain and cut off the blood supply to the area. The cells in the area that don't get blood flow, die off and cause damage. How big an area that blood vessel feeds determines the extent of damage, as well as how big the blockage is, how long it lasts, and how many cells die. If your clot is dissolved quickly and few or no cells die, this is called a TIA, or transient ischemic attack. However, if blood flow is not restored within six minutes, cells die and cause damage and loss of function. This is called a stroke. The same process can occur in your heart and you get a heart attack, otherwise known as a myocardial infarction. It can happen in your kidneys or any other part of your body.

What Is Ischemia?

If plaque buildup occurs and narrows the arteries in your legs, it is called peripheral artery disease (PAD). Your need for more oxygen supplied by blood flow through your arteries is increased when you walk, yet the arteries are narrow, and your muscles do not get the amount of blood flow needed to supply the demand, causing pain. This pain is called ischemia. The same ischemia occurs as a warning sign if blood flow is diminished in your heart. It can be sensed as chest tightness or pressure, numbness in your arm or jaw, nausea, shortness of breath, or vague symptoms of indigestion. However, in some people there is a sudden breakup of plaque that is large, and a heart attack or stroke can occur suddenly without any warning.

You can see why having clear, elastic arteries is important to maintain overall health. The arterial system is the source of the nutrients and oxygen that keep cells alive and functioning optimally. They also maintain the flow and pressure needed for changes in activity level and position. The plaque not only changes the elasticity, but it also changes the flow. Let's look at some of the factors that contribute to the development of plaque formation, and the development of cardiovascular disease and all its complications.

Risk Factors for Cardiovascular Disease

One risk factor may not be enough to develop outright disease, and all risk factors are not created equal. Some risk factors can be more easily managed than others, and some carry more weight than others. Each risk factor can have an additive effect, which can be more than the sum of its parts. In the case of cholesterol, we label subtypes of cholesterol as independent risk factors, which means that even if the total cholesterol is normal, an elevation in any one of the sub-types that is an independent risk factor. We can have one or more risk factors related to lipids even if the cholesterol is normal. We look at each risk factor independently. Here are some modifiable and non-modifiable risk factors:

- Age
- Male sex
- Family history or race
- Smoking

- High cholesterol
- High blood pressure
- Overweight or obese
- Diabetes

Fat Facts and the Faces of Cholesterol

The National Heart, Blood and Lung Institute states that over 50% of people with heart attacks have normal cholesterol. It's not just the amount of cholesterol you have; it's the size and type of particles that determine your risk. Cholesterol is a group of lipids characterized by their density such as high density lipoprotein (HDL), low density lipoprotein (LDL), and very low density lipoprotein (VLDL) and triglycerides. Cholesterol screening tests calculate your low density lipoprotein (LDL) and don't actually measure the amount or size of your LDL particles. Advanced lipoprotein particle testing and testing for other risk factors can give you a more complete picture.

Particle Size or Density, and Number

A measured LDL can give you a better picture of your risk. The size makes a difference and contributes to risk. The smaller the particle, the more likely it will get oxidized, lodge between the cells in the arteries, and cause damage. Just think how easy it would be for small particles to squeeze between cells and lodge there. A large particle would more likely bounce off, get carried off in your bloodstream, and be used to make hormones or cell walls.

Measured LDL	Particle Size	Particle Number
160 mg/dl	Very Large	20
160 mg/dl	Large	40
160 mg/dl	Small	80
160 mg/dl	Very Small	160

Small and dense (regardless of type) are more easily lodged in the artery walls, causing inflammation and plaque formation.

Particle Type

When you eat something with fat in it, it is carried through your bloodstream in packets called chylomicrons that have a mix of fats, such as triglycerides and cholesterol, and proteins, such as lipoproteins and apo proteins. The lipoproteins allow fat, which is not dissolved in blood, to be carried through to your cells, tissues, and organs that need it for growth and repair.

As chylomicrons travel through your bloodstream, the fats are broken down, and some fat and protein are removed and taken up by cells for energy. The removal of these changes the density and composition of the packets from very low density (VLDL) to intermediate density (IDL, or remnant particle) to low density (LDL). Each particle (VLDL, IDL, LDL) has a function and is a risk factor for cardiovascular disease.

Advanced Testing: Lipoprotein Particle Analysis

- **High density lipoprotein (HDL):** HDL transports cholesterol back to the liver. We want HDL to be high. This can be accomplished through exercising, maintaining an ideal weight, not smoking, and taking medications and supplements such as statins, niacin, fibrates, and/or estrogen, and drinking moderate amounts of alcohol.

- **Low density lipoprotein (LDL):** Small dense particles are most likely to get oxidized, inflamed, form plaque and clots, and cause damage to artery walls. Fluffing up the particles and making them larger reduces the risk of damage. Particle size can be increased with Omega 3 fatty acids in fish and other oils, and the number of particles can be decreased with decreasing the saturated fats in your diet, exercise, niacin, statins, and other types of cholesterol-lowering drugs, as well as estrogen.

- **Intermediate density lipoprotein (IDL) or remnant particles (RP):** This is an independent risk factor because these particles don't need to be oxidized to cause damage. White blood cells called macrophages swallow these up, and then the macrophage becomes a foam cell, which send signals to cause inflammation and plaque formation. It bypasses the process of oxidation that is needed for LDL to cause the same process. Many of the same things that lower triglycerides lower LDL.

- **Triglycerides (TG):** Triglycerides are also an independent risk factor for cardiovascular disease. They are lowered by diet, especially by decreasing sugar, alcohol, refined carbohydrates, and saturated fat. Other things that lower triglycerides are exercise, statins, niacin, and other cholesterol-lowering drugs, and Omega 3 fatty acids.

- **Lipoprotein (a) (Lp (a)):** This is an independent risk factor for developing cardiovascular disease and carries more weight than LDL cholesterol. Not only is it smaller and denser, it is more easily oxidized, causing inflammation, and promotes the formation of clots narrowing the blood vessels. As we know, clots on top of plaque break off and cause blockages in the arteries. Although genetics determine the amount to some extent, you can modify it by correcting estrogen deficiency and supplementing with niacin.

The table on the next page is an example of some of the factors that have an effect on the various types of cholesterol. You can better tailor treatment based on particle types, which is why I recommend consulting an anti-aging metabolic specialist.

Particle	Diet & Exercise	Niacin	Statins	Omega 3	Estrogen	Other
HDL	Exercise Moderate alcohol Low glycemic	X	X	--------	X	No Smoking Ideal Weight Fibrates
LDL	Low saturated fat	X	X	Increases particle size not number	X	Resins Fibrates Absorption Inhibitors
RP & TG	Low glycemic	X	X	X	--------	Absorption Inhibitors
Lp(a)	--------	X	--------	--------	X	--------

You can see that just measuring cholesterol by standard means leaves out part of the picture, and it's not as simple as good and bad cholesterol. The good cholesterol can be bad if the particles are small and dense, and the bad cholesterol can be tamed if the particles are larger and fluffier. Recent studies indicate that niacin is as effective as statin drugs in reducing cholesterol; however, flushing can be an issue. This flushing can be managed and the dose of niacin lowered by using a combination of aspirin and other nutrients. Niacin raises HDL substantially and also may beneficially alter total cholesterol, LDL, and triglyceride levels. Niacin also exhibits antioxidant, anti-inflammatory, and other beneficial effects on hardening of the arteries or atherosclerosis. Treatment can be tailored based on particle types, numbers, and size, diet, hormones, weight, and other factors.

Know your numbers. Knowledge is power, and you have the power to change your numbers with nutrients and diet. These tests cost a bit more than a traditional cholesterol screening test and may be covered by insurance. Some laboratories package these to make it affordable. Knowing your numbers enables you and your doctor to tailor the treatment to your specific needs.

Customize Cholesterol Control and Other Factors

An advanced test can measure your particle types and sizes so treatment can be customized for you. Biomarkers can tell you where you have a breakdown in the process. Genetic testing will give us an understanding of how your enzymes and genes will react to drugs, supplements, and dietary and environmental factors, and functional micronutrient testing will give more specific guidelines regarding how to dose supplements.

Beyond the Basics Biomarkers

It is important to look at all of the parts of the process of developing cardiovascular and other related diseases and risk factors. Let's look at what we can learn from biomarkers in customizing an approach to managing cardiovascular disease, risk factors, and other diseases.

- **C-Reactive Protein (CRP):** a biomarker of inflammation. Many of the degenerative diseases of aging could be attributed to inflammation. These include everything from allergies, Alzheimer's, arthritis, autoimmune disease, cancer, and more.
  - o Inflammation can be modulated by your diet, as discussed in Chapter 2, and nutrients that quiet inflammation. These include but are not limited to: boswellia, bromelain, chondroitin, curcumin, fish oils, ginger, glucosamine, grape-seed extract, green tea, pycnogenol, quercetin, and turmeric. Since oxidation causes inflammation, antioxidants such as alpha lipoic acid, glutathione, N acetyl cysteine, and Vitamins A, C, and E can be helpful.
- **Homocysteine:** a biomarker for metabolism of folic acid metabolism. A high homocysteine level is a risk factor for cardiovascular disease. It damages blood vessel walls, leading to high blood pressure, peripheral artery disease, stroke, elevated cholesterol and triglycerides, and Alzheimer's disease.
  - o Homocysteine is a risk factor for brain atrophy, cognitive impairment, and dementia. Plasma con-

centrations of homocysteine can be lowered by dietary administration of B vitamins. It promotes free radical production, which leads to oxidation and cell death.

o You can lower homocysteine by giving Vitamins B6 and B12 and folate, exercising, and replenishing estrogen if it is low. Some people have a genetic reason for high levels because of a reduction in the 5, 10-methylenetetrahydrofolate reductase (MTHFR) enzyme that metabolizes folate. If this is the case, they need an activated form of folate as well as methyl groups such as betaine or trimethylglycine.

- **Fasting Insulin:** a biomarker for insulin sensitivity and an indicator of pre-diabetes, diabetes, or metabolic syndrome. Insulin affects the ability of glucose to get into cells as well as fat storage. Glucose is required for fuel and energy. The receptors that recognize insulin and make it work can sometimes stop recognizing insulin, causing your body to keep making more insulin.

  o Excess insulin elevates blood lipids and blood sugar, and makes an enzyme that tells your body to make androgens instead of estrogen. (That is why women with polycystic ovarian syndrome (PCOS) have increased facial hair. Insulin resistance is part of the syndrome.) Cardiovascular disease and diabetes are linked to insulin resistance.

  o Alpha lipoic acid, chromium, cinnamon, plant extracts from hops and acacia, Omega 3 fatty acids, and Vitamin D can enhance insulin sensitivity.

  o Inflammation is also a contributor to insulin resistance, as are being overweight and sedentary. Any factors that modulate inflammation and weight will have a positive effect on insulin sensitivity. Aging also contributes to insulin resistance and, although we will all age, we can slow the metabolic processes that contribute to accelerated aging.

- **Hemoglobin A1C:** a biomarker for sugar bound to protein. When excess sugar binds to proteins, this is like throwing a monkey wrench into your system. The process of sugar binding to proteins is called glycation, which changes the protein's function. An example of glycation is a cataract. Sugar binds to protein in the lens of your eye and makes it cloudy. It doesn't function well. Since these proteins are building blocks of all cells and tissues and allow for regeneration and repair, this process of glycation accelerates aging.

  o Diabetics are more prone to complications because they have excess sugar and glycation occurs in every organ in the body. A low glycemic diet and factors that regulate inflammation and insulin sensitivity may also have an effect.

Functional Micronutrient Testing

We saw from Chapter 3 that nutrient deficiencies are prevalent and may be implicated in many diseases. Cardiovascular disease and metabolic syndrome, which increases the risk of diabetes and other diseases, are associated with deficiencies in alpha lipoic acid, chromium, Vitamin B12, Vitamin B6, folate, and antioxidants, as well as magnesium, coenzyme Q10 (Co Q10), otherwise known as ubiquinone, and selenium. While we can test the blood levels, we may know if the nutrients are being absorbed and circulating. We may not know whether they enter the cells and are having the desired affect. There are unique methods to determine if you have cellular deficiencies and the dose of nutrients needed to correct them. This is truly a great way to customize your supplement recommendations. These would be offered by metabolic, functional medicine, and anti-aging specialists, but are not readily available through your family doctor or primary care physician. In Chapter 3, we discussed the variety of nutritional deficiencies that are prevalent, and this is an easy and relatively inexpensive way to test about thirty-three nutrients.

Cardiogenomics

Genetic testing can be quite valuable to determine response to drugs, nutrients, and lifestyle interventions. Here are examples of some common genetic variants and their associated illnesses:

- **Apolipoprotein E (APO-E)** removes cholesterol from the blood-stream. There are several genetic variants, which act differently. The variant called APO-E4 has a tendency toward higher levels of LDL and lower levels of HDL, and therefore increases the risk of hardening of the arteries with plaque, heart attack, and stroke. Statin drugs don't work as well in APO-E4 carriers, and estrogen replacement can be beneficial. It has also been implicated in Alzheimer's disease.

- **Methylenetetrahydrofolate reductase (MTHFR)** is a key enzyme in folate metabolism. This was mentioned in relation to homocysteine. Two variants of the MTHFR polymorphisms result in reduced enzyme activity and increased risk of cardiovascular disease, stroke, abdominal aortic aneurysm, hypertension, and blood clots in your veins. We can manage this process by giving an activated form of folic acid called methyl tetra hydro folate, or MTHF, and methyl donors such as betaine or trimethylglycine, as well as extra B vitamins such as B2, B3, B6, and B12.

- **Factor II** is also known as prothrombin. Prothrombin is a protein in blood that gets transformed into thrombin and aids in blood clotting. Variants or polymorphisms of Factor II result in increased blood clotting, especially in your veins. Prothrombin is also associated with increased risk of cardiovascular disease, carotid atherosclerosis, atrial fibrillation, and MI (when other cardiovascular risk factors are present).

- **Factor V (Leiden)** is the gene variant that affects the conversion of prothrombin to thrombin and increases the risk for clotting and coronary artery disease. If you have the SNPs in Factor II or MTHFR, it has an additive effect making the clotting worse.

The standard of care is just that: It is the standard that fits most people. However, you are unique, and if you are not in the middle of the bell-shaped curve and the standard doesn't work, you can be left frustrated and not get the full benefit of treatment options.

You can manage your cholesterol and other metabolic processes of aging and illness with the basic synergistic strategies of diet, exercise, supplements, and stress management, or take it to another level with a deeper look at your unique metabolic and genetic makeup and a customized fitness, nutrition, and supplement program that takes all of your unique nuances into consideration. A metabolic, anti-aging specialist can dig deeper; perform functional, metabolic, and genetic tests; and customize a program and take out the guesswork.

Some people may require more supplements than others. The number of supplements to take can be overwhelming. Buying many bottles of supplements with redundant ingredients that can leave you with overdosing on nutrients you don't need, as well as under-dosing the nutrients you do need, may not be the best solution. You can have a formula custom-manufactured to your specific needs so you get the exact amount you need in one package. This makes it easy to travel and order (because you always run out of some things before others).

We used cardiovascular disease as an example of what to look for and how to customize treatment based on test results. However, the same methods can be applied to other illnesses, such as osteoporosis, diabetes, and cancer. It's a matter of looking at the process of how the condition develops, checking the biomarkers, looking for deficiencies, and modulating the genetic factors that contribute.

Beyond the Basics Testing Recommendations

You may benefit from some or all of the following tests based on your symptoms, history, family history, and lifestyle. A metabolic or anti-aging specialist can help you determine which may be most beneficial.

- Lipoprotein particle analysis
- C-Reactive protein (CRP)

- Homocysteine
- Fasting insulin
- Hemoglobin A1C
- Functional micronutrient testing
- Organic acids
- Genomic testing
- Hormone testing
- Hormone metabolites

You have entered the new age of medicine. A true preventive approach and a paradigm shift. Harnessing the synergistic power of nutrition, supplements, exercise, hormones, and advanced testing can allow you to live younger and healthier. Live, love, laugh, and enjoy life with health and vigor.

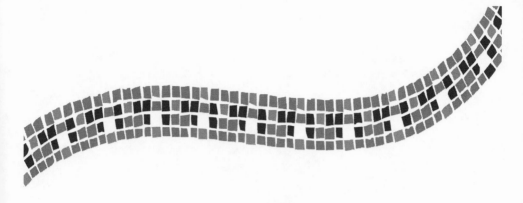

Appendix I

Workbook

Getting Ready: Assess

Where am I now?

- What am I most afraid of?

- What is bothering me the most?

- If I changed one thing, what would make the most difference in my life?

Where do I want to go?

- What does it look and feel like to reach my goal?

- Why do I want this?

- What is my ultimate goal?

- Do I want to start small or get to the bottom of all of my issues more quickly?

- What am I willing to do to reach my goal?

Getting Set: Plan

Create a Vision

What will it look and feel like when I improve or reach my goals?

My vision for my life and health are:

Achieving this vision will impact my life in the following ways:
- Physical

- Emotional

- Financial

- Social

- Other

SMART Goals (Specific, Measurable, Attainable, Realistic, Time Bound)

- Food choices
- Supplements
- Exercise

- Hormone balance
- Stress management
- Other

Go: Action!

- Height
- Weight
- Blood pressure
- Pulse
- Body mass index (BMI)
- Body composition (percent fat)
- Waist size
- Hip size
- Waist-to-hip ratio
- Fasting blood sugar
- Metabolic panel or chem. screen
- Complete blood count (CBC)
- Lipids (total cholesterol, LDL, HDL, and triglycerides)

Age- or gender-specific tests:

- Prostate specific antigen (PSA)
- Pap smear
- Mammography

- DEXA bone scan
- Hormone levels

Advanced testing:

- Lipoprotein particle analysis
- C- Reactive Protein (CRP)
- Homocysteine
- Fasting insulin
- Hemoglobin A1c

Beyond the basic tests:

- Metabolic testing
- Genetic testing
- Other

Based on my risk factors, numbers, and family history, my next steps are:

1.
2.
3.
4.
5.
6.
7.
8.
9.
10.

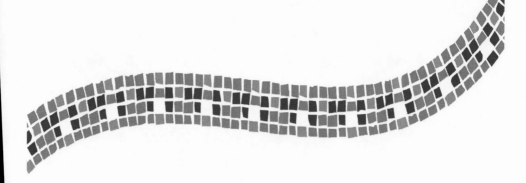

Appendix II

Additional Reference Tables

Blood Pressure

Systolic (mm Hg)	Diastolic (mm Hg)	Risk for Cardiovascular Disease
120 or less	80 or less	Very low
121 – 130	81 – 85	Low
131 – 140	86 – 90	Moderate
141 – 150	91 – 100	High
151 or greater	101 or greater	Very High

Adapted from the National Heart, Lung and Blood Institute Diseases and Conditions Index.

Body Mass Index (BMI)

BMI	19	20	21	22	23	24	25	26	27	28	29	30	36	40
Height	Weight													
58	91	96	100	105	110	115	119	124	129	134	138	143	167	191
59	94	99	104	109	114	119	124	128	133	138	143	148	173	198
60	97	102	107	112	118	123	128	133	138	143	148	153	179	204
61	100	106	111	116	122	127	132	137	143	148	153	158	185	211
62	104	109	115	120	126	131	136	142	147	153	158	164	191	218
63	107	113	118	124	130	135	141	146	152	158	163	169	197	225
64	107	113	118	124	130	135	141	146	152	158	163	169	197	225
65	114	120	126	132	138	144	150	156	162	168	174	180	210	240
66	118	124	130	136	142	148	155	161	167	173	179	186	216	247
67	121	127	134	140	146	153	159	166	172	178	185	191	223	225
68	128	135	142	149	155	162	169	176	182	189	196	203	236	270
69	128	135	142	149	155	162	169	176	182	189	196	203	236	270
70	132	139	146	153	160	167	174	181	188	195	202	207	243	278
71	136	143	150	157	165	172	179	186	193	200	208	215	250	286
72	140	147	154	162	169	177	184	191	199	206	213	221	258	294
73	144	151	159	166	174	182	189	197	204	212	219	227	265	302
74	148	155	163	171	179	186	194	202	210	218	225	233	272	311
75	152	160	168	176	184	192	200	208	216	224	232	240	279	319
76	156	164	172	180	189	197	205	213	221	230	238	246	287	328

Adapted from the National Heart, Lung and Blood Institute, Classification of Overweight and Obesity by BMI, Waist Circumference and Associated Disease Risk.

BMI Classification

BMI	Class	Waist Men < 40" or 102 cm Women < 30" or 88 cm	Waist Men > 102" Women > 88"
18.5 or less	Underweight	-	-
18.5 – 24.9	Normal	-	-
25.0 – 29.9	Overweight	Increased	High
30.0 – 34.9	Obese	High	Very High
35.0 – 39.9	Obese	Very High	Very High
40.0 or more	Extremely Obese	Extremely High	Extremely High

Adapted from the National Heart, Lung and Blood Institute, Classification of Overweight and Obesity by BMI, Waist Circumference and Associated Disease Risk.

Cholesterol

Goals for LDL Based on Risk Factors for Coronary Heart Disease	
Coronary Heart Disease	< 100 mg/dl
2 or more risk factors for CHD	<130 mg/dl
0-1 Risk factor	< 160 mg/dl

Adapted from the National Heart, Lung and Blood Institute: Detection, Evaluation and Treatment of High Blood Cholesterol in Adults ATP III Final Report.

HDL	
Good	> 60 mg/dl
Too low	< 40 mg/dl

Triglycerides	
Normal	<150 mg/dl
Borderline	150 – 199 mg/dl
High	200 – 499 mg/dl
Very High	≥ 500 mg/dl

Adapted from the National Heart, Lung and Blood Institute: Detection, Evaluation and Treatment of High Blood Cholesterol in Adults ATP III Final Report.

Blood Tests for Diabetes and Insulin Resistance

	Fasting Blood Sugar	Hemoglobin A1C (HbA1C)	Fasting Insulin Units =iUI/ml
Ideal	65 – 86 mg/dl	< 5%	<6 iUI/ml
Normal	<100 mg/dl	< 6%	6-27 iUI/ml
Pre-diabetes	100-125 mg/dl	> 6%	>15 Insulin Resistance
Diabetes	> 126 mg/dl	>7%	

Compiled and adapted from "A Comprehensive Guide to Preventive Blood Testing" (*Life Extension Magazine*, May 2004), and "Aging and Glycation" (*Life Extension Magazine*, April 2008).

Other Biomarkers of Risk

	Homocysteine Umol/l	C-reactive protein mg/dl	Fibrinogen mg/dl
Optimal	< 7	< 0.55	200 – 300 mg/dl
Good	< 10 good	< 0.7	200 – 400 mg/dl
Normal	5 – 15 Normal	< 1	

Adapted from "A Comprehensive Guide to Preventive Blood Testing" (*Life Extension Magazine*, May 2004).

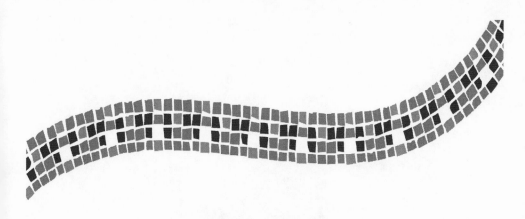

Appendix III

Nutrition Tracking Worksheet

The most effective way to monitor your intake and track your progress it to write down what you eat on a daily basis. Most people don't remember what they ate unless they write it down. Use the tracking sheet as a guide to record your intake so you can determine if you are eating balanced meals and to monitor the quality and portion sizes to improve your health.

Date	Lean Protein (palm of hand)	Complex Carbohydrate (fist if Glycemic Index <70; half-fist if high glycemic; 2 fists for leafy vegetables)	Unsaturated Fat (4 dice; 1 T.)	Fluids	List foods that are not in this category
Breakfast Within an hour of waking **Rainbow of colors**					
Snack 1 4 – 5 hours after last meal **Rainbow of colors**					
Lunch 4 – 5 hours after last meal **Rainbow of colors**					
Snack 2 4 – 5 hours after last meal **Rainbow of colors**					
Dinner At least 4 hours before bedtime **Rainbow of colors**					

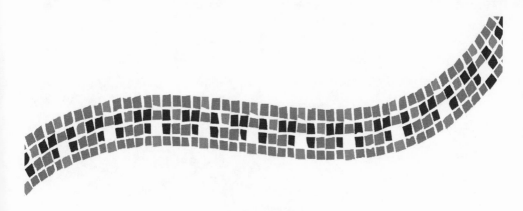

Appendix IV

Elimination Diet

The elimination diet can help you heal as well as determine if you have any sensitivities or intolerances to foods. Combining this with supplements and herbs to help your liver process and eliminate toxins can unmask hidden sensitivities, quiet your immune system, and relieve symptoms that may be caused by foods, additives, preservatives, herbicides, pesticides, and other chemicals.

Eliminate processed foods that have dyes, additives, preservatives, and artificial ingredients. Any meats or poultry must be grass-fed, hormone-free, and organic. Fruits and vegetables from the dirty dozen must be organic. (The "dirty dozen" are foods with the highest amount of pesticide residues: peaches, apples, sweet bell peppers, celery, nectarines, strawberries, cherries, pears, grapes, spinach, lettuce, and potatoes.)

Drink filtered or purified water, and use filtered water for coffee and tea.

The following is a modified version. If you don't get relief of symptoms, you may need to eliminate more and follow a stricter version.

Food Group	Allowed	Avoid
Meat, Fish, Poultry	Chicken, turkey, lamb, legumes, dried peas and lentils, cold-water fish (salmon, halibut, and mackerel)	Red meats, cold cuts, frankfurters, canned meats, eggs, shellfish, soy products
Dairy	Milk substitutes such as rice and nut milks	Milk, cheese, ice cream, cream, non-dairy creamers
Starch	Sweet potato, rice, tapioca, buckwheat, and gluten-free products	All gluten-containing products, bread, pasta, corn
Soups	Clear, vegetable-based broth; homemade vegetarian soups	Canned or creamed soups
Vegetables	All vegetables except corn and potatoes (preferably fresh, frozen, or freshly juiced)	Creamed vegetables, vegetables in casseroles, corn, canned vegetables with sauce, soy products

Food Group	Allowed	Avoid
Beverages	Unsweetened fruit or vegetable juices, water, non-citrus herbal tea	Milk, coffee, tea, cocoa, alcoholic beverages, soda, sweetened beverages, artificial sweeteners except stevia, citrus, soy
Bread, Cereals, and Grains	Rice, buckwheat, millet, soy, potato, tapioca, arrowroot, or gluten-free oats	Wheat, oat, spelt, kamut, rye, barley, or other gluten-containing products (NOTE: Some oats are cross-contaminated with gluten.)
Fruit	Unsweetened fresh or frozen fruits, except citrus and strawberries	Fruit drinks, citrus, strawberries, dried fruit, sweetened canned fruit
Fats, Oil, and Nuts	Cold expeller pressed unrefined oils: canola, flax, olive, or sunflower oil, ghee, sesame; seeds: sesame, flax, pumpkin, squash; nuts: almonds, cashews, pecans, walnuts	Margarine, shortening, unclarified butter, refined oils, peanuts, store-bought salad dressings and spreads, hydrogenated oil, cooking sprays, mayonnaise

Try as best you can to eliminate all toxins, such as the following.

Environmental:

- Air pollution
- Auto exhaust
- Solvents (paints, cleaning products, etc.)
- Heavy metals
- Pesticides
- Herbicides
- Insecticides
- Radiation
- Inhalants

Lifestyle:

- Nicotine
- Alcohol
- Caffeine
- Drugs
- Meats that contain hormones and antibiotics
- Artificial food additives, coloring, and preservatives
- Refined foods and sugars
- Fast food
- Fried food

After two to four weeks, or when you feel good, introduce foods one at a time every three days. Eat the foods you are introducing two or three times in the same day. Do not introduce any new foods over the two days that follow. Always go back to the baseline diet. For example when adding eggs, eat two or three meals a day with some egg for two to three days, and write down your symptoms for three days. Stop eating eggs after the third day and introduce wheat. Whenever you add a new food, don't mix with any other foods that are not on the elimination diet. Just add one food at a time, as some foods may interact with each other.

Write down the food you introduced and any reactions. Note if you experience digestive or bowel issues, such as bloating, gas, constipation, abdominal pain, or diarrhea, headache, nasal congestion or mucous, skin reactions such as redness or itching, changes in energy, mood, or mental clarity, joint or muscle aches or pains, and any other symptoms. If any reactions occur, eliminate the food for three months before re-introducing it. Oftentimes, a temporary break from a food will allow you to tolerate it in moderation. Rotate foods every four days to avoid intolerances.

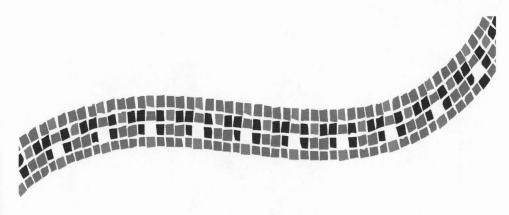

Appendix V

Fitness

Calculate Your Heart Rate

- Maximum Heart Rate (220 – age) = MHR
  My MHR is _____.
- Target Heart Rate THR 65–85% MHR
  My target zone is _____.

- If de-conditioned, determine what your heart rate is when you can talk but not sing while doing an aerobic activity.
- My comfort zone HR is _____.

Tracking Sheets

Use the Resistance Exercise and Cardio Endurance tracking sheets to record your workout activity and to track your progress.

Resistance Exercise Tracking Sheet

Week:	Date		Date		Date		Date		Date		Date		Date		Date	
Exercise	Wt.	Reps	Wt.	Reps	Wt.	Reps	Wt.	Reps	Wt.	Reps	Wt.	Reps	Wt.	Reps	Wt.	Reps
Quads/Glutes																
Hamstrings																
Chest																
Back																
Shoulders																
Biceps																
Triceps																
Calves																
Low Back																
Abdominals																

Cardio Endurance Tracking Sheet

Date	Monday		Tuesday		Wednesday		Thursday		Friday		Saturday		Sunday	
Type	Time	THR	Time	THR	Time	THR	Time	THR	Time	THR	Time	THR	Time	THR

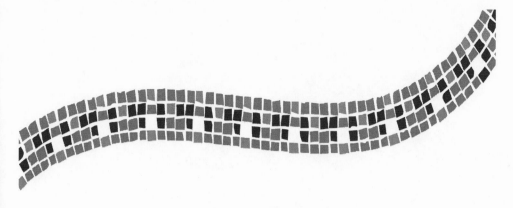

Appendix VI

Hormone Harmony

Managing Insulin and Cortisol Through Diet

List your favorite low-glycemic foods.

List your favorite anti-inflammatory foods.

List all the different colored fruits and vegetables that are low glycemic that you like.

(Include foods that you are not sure if you would like but are willing to try.)

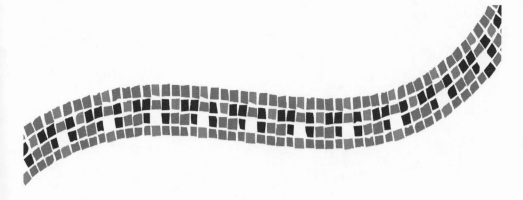

Appendix VII

Stress Management

What situations do I find stressful?

How can I better manage these situations?

How can I respond better to these situations?

What stress-management techniques would be useful in these situations?

What stress-management techniques am I willing to practice

(e.g., breath work, progressive muscle relaxation, meditation, exercise, laughter, music, saying no, yoga)?

What am I grateful for?

Who do I need to forgive?

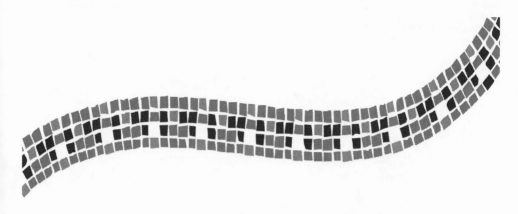

References

Chapter 1: Get Motivated

Eccles, Jacquelynne S., and Allan Wigfield. "Motivational beliefs, values, and goals." *Annual Review of Psychology* 53 (2002): 109–132.

Locke, Edwin A., and Gary P. Latham. "Building a practically useful theory of goal setting and task motivation. A 35-year odyssey." *The American Psychologist* 57, no. 9 (September 2002): 705–717.

Potempa, Kathleen M., Susan W. Butterworth, Marna K. Flaherty-Robb, and William L. Gaynor. "The Healthy Ageing Model: health behaviour change for older adults." *Collegian (Royal College of Nursing, Australia)* 17, no. 2 (2010): 51–55.

Ryan, Polly. "Integrated Theory of Health Behavior Change: background and intervention development." *Clinical Nurse Specialist* 23, no. 3 (June 2009): 161–170; quiz 171–172.

Chapter 2: Food as Medicine

Anderle, Pascale, Pierre Farmer, Alvin Berger, and Matthew Alan Roberts. "Nutrigenomic approach to understanding the mechanisms by which dietary long-chain fatty acids induce gene signals and control mechanisms involved in carcinogenesis." *Nutrition (Burbank, Los Angeles County, Calif.)* 20, no. 1 (January 2004): 103–108.

Anderson, J.A. "Food allergy and food intolerance." *ASDC Journal of Dentistry for Children* 52, no. 2 (April 1985): 134–137.

Barclay, Alan W., Peter Petocz, Joanna McMillan-Price, Victoria M. Flood, Tania Prvan, Paul Mitchell, and Jennie C. Brand-Miller. "Glycemic index, glycemic load, and chronic disease risk—a meta-analysis of observational studies." *The American Journal of Clinical Nutrition* 87, no. 3 (March 2008): 627–637.

Björntorp, P. "Abdominal fat distribution and disease: an overview of epidemiological data." *Annals of Medicine* 24, no. 1 (February 1992): 15–18.

Blades, Mabel. *The Glycemic Load Counter: A Pocket Guide to GL and GI Values for over 800 Foods.* Ulysses Press, 2008.

Bonora, Enzo. "Postprandial peaks as a risk factor for cardiovascular disease: epidemiological perspectives." *International Journal of Clinical Practice. Supplement,* no. 129 (July 2002): 5–11.

Bourre, J.M. "Effects of nutrients (in food) on the structure and function of the nervous system: update on dietary requirements for brain. Part 2: macronutrients." *The Journal of Nutrition, Health & Aging* 10, no. 5 (October 2006): 386–399.

———. "Roles of unsaturated fatty acids (especially omega-3 fatty acids) in the brain at various ages and during ageing." *The Journal of Nutrition, Health & Aging* 8, no. 3 (2004): 163–174.

Brod, S.A. "Unregulated inflammation shortens human functional longevity." *Inflammation Research: Official Journal of the European Histamine Research Society ... [et al]* 49, no. 11 (November 2000): 561–570.

Carey, V.J., E.E. Walters, G.A. Colditz, C.G. Solomon, W.C. Willett, B.A. Rosner, F.E. Speizer, and J.E. Manson. "Body fat distribution and risk of non-insulin-dependent diabetes mellitus in women. The Nurses' Health Study." *American Journal of Epidemiology* 145, no. 7 (April 1, 1997): 614–619.

Carlsen, Monica H., Bente L. Halvorsen, Kari Holte, Siv K. Bøhn, Steinar Dragland, Laura Sampson, Carol Willey, et al. "The total antioxidant content of more than 3100 foods, beverages, spices, herbs and supplements used worldwide." *Nutrition Journal* 9 (2010): 3.

Carroccio, Antonio, Lidia Di Prima, Giuseppe Iacono, Ada M. Florena, Francesco D'Arpa, Carmelo Sciumè, Angelo B. Cefalù, Davide Noto, and Maurizio R. Averna. "Multiple food hypersensitivity as a cause of refractory chronic constipation in adults." *Scandinavian Journal of Gastroenterology* 41, no. 4 (April 2006): 498–504.

Ch'ng, Chin Lye, M. Keston Jones, and Jeremy G.C. Kingham. "Celiac disease and autoimmune thyroid disease." *Clinical Medicine & Research* 5, no. 3 (October 2007): 184–192.

Decaterina, R. "n-3 Fatty acids and the inflammatory response — biological background." *European Heart Journal Supplements* 3 (6, 2001): D42–D49.

Draper, Mark. "How diet has changed over 70 years." *Nutrition and the Environment,* June 2001.

Drisko, Jeanne, Bette Bischoff, Matthew Hall, and Richard McCallum. "Treating irritable bowel syndrome with a food elimination diet followed by food challenge and probiotics." *Journal of the American College of Nutrition* 25, no. 6 (December 2006): 514–522.

"Drugs & Supplements: Omega-3 fatty acids, fish oil, alpha-linolenic acid (Print Version)," May 3, 2006.

Eaton, S.B., S.B. Eaton, and M.J. Konner. "Paleolithic nutrition revisited: a twelve-year retrospective on its nature and implications." *European Journal of Clinical Nutrition* 51, no. 4 (April 1997): 207–216.

Eaton, S.B., and M. Konner. "Paleolithic nutrition. A consideration of its nature and current implications." *The New England Journal of Medicine* 312, no. 5 (January 31, 1985): 283–289.

Finck, Brian N. "Effects of PPARalpha on cardiac glucose metabolism: a transcriptional equivalent of the glucose-fatty acid cycle?" *Expert Review of Cardiovascular Therapy* 4, no. 2 (March 2006): 161–171.

———. "The role of the peroxisome proliferator-activated receptor alpha pathway in pathological remodeling of the diabetic heart." *Current Opinion in Clinical Nutrition and Metabolic Care* 7, no. 4 (July 2004): 391–396.

Fontana, Luigi. "The scientific basis of caloric restriction leading to longer life." *Current Opinion in Gastroenterology* 25, no. 2 (March 2009): 144–150.

Fritsche, Kevin. "Fatty acids as modulators of the immune response." *Annual Review of Nutrition* 26, no. 1 (8, 2006): 45–73.

Furst, Peter, and Peter Stehle. "What are the essential elements needed for the determination of amino acid requirements in humans?" *The Journal of Nutrition.* 134, no. 6 (June 1, 2004): 1558S–1565.

Geberhiwot, Tarekegn, Angela Haddon, and Mourad Labib. "HbA1c predicts the likelihood of having impaired glucose tolerance in high-risk patients with normal fasting plasma glucose." *Annals of Clinical Biochemistry* 42, no. 3 (May 2005): 193–195.

Genuis, Stephen J. "Sensitivity-related illness: The escalating pandemic of allergy, food intolerance and chemical sensitivity." *The Science of the Total Environment* (October 2, 2010). www.ncbi.nlm.nih.gov/pubmed/20920818.

"Glycemic index and glycemic load for 100+ foods." *Harvard Health Publications*, n.d. www.health.harvard.edu/newsweek/ Glycemic_index_and_glycemic_load_for_100_foods.htm.

Gorman, Christine. "The fires within." *Time*, February 23, 2004.

Gray, D.S., and K. Fujioka. "Use of relative weight and body mass index for the determination of adiposity." *Journal of Clinical Epidemiology* 44, no. 6 (1991): 545–550.

Gray, D.S., K. Fujioka, W. Devine, and T. Cuyegkeng. "Abdominal obesity is associated with insulin resistance." *Family Medicine* 25, no. 6 (June 1993): 396–400.

Harper, A.E. "Some comments on protein and amino acid utilization." *The American Journal of Clinical Nutrition* 11 (November 1962): 382–388.

Hoffman, Jay R. "Protein—which is best?" *Journal of Sports Sciend and Medicine* 3 (n.d.): 118–130.

Huang, Wu-Yang, Yi-Zhong Cai, and Yanbo Zhang. "Natural phenolic compounds from medicinal herbs and dietary plants: potential use for cancer prevention." *Nutrition and Cancer* 62, no. 1 (2010): 1–20.

Hurrell, Richard F. "Influence of vegetable protein sources on trace element and mineral bioavailability." *The Journal of Nutrition* 133, no. 9 (September 2003): 2973S–7S.

Jarisch, R., and F. Wantke. "Wine and headache." *International Archives of Allergy and Immunology* 110, no. 1 (May 1996): 7–12.

Jump, Donald B. "Fatty acid regulation of gene transcription." *Critical Reviews in Clinical Laboratory Sciences* 41, no. 1 (2004): 41–78.

Kreider, Richard B., and Bill Campbell. "Protein for exercise and recovery." *The Physician and Sportsmedicine* 37, no. 2 (June 2009): 13–21.

Kris-Etherton, P.M., D.S. Taylor, S. Yu-Poth, P. Huth, K. Moriarty, V. Fishell, R.L. Hargrove, G. Zhao, and T.D. Etherton. "Polyunsaturated fatty acids in the food chain in the United States." *The American Journal of Clinical Nutrition* 71, no. 1 (January 2000): 179S–88S.

Krishnan, Supriya, Lynn Rosenberg, Martha Singer, Frank B. Hu, Luc Djoussé, L. Adrienne Cupples, and Julie R. Palmer. "Glycemic index, glycemic load, and cereal fiber intake and risk of type 2 diabetes in US black women." *Archives of Internal Medicine* 167, no. 21 (November 26, 2007): 2304–2309.

Kumar, V., M. Rajadhyaksha, and J. Wortsman. "Celiac disease-associated autoimmune endocrinopathies." *Clinical and Diagnostic Laboratory Immunology* 8, no. 4 (July 2001): 678–685.

Kwon, Dae Young, James W. Daily, Hyun Jin Kim, and Sunmin Park. "Antidiabetic effects of fermented soybean products on type 2 diabetes." *Nutrition Research (New York, N.Y.)* 30, no. 1 (January 2010): 1–13.

Larsen, Clark Spencer. "Animal source foods and human health during evolution." *The Journal of Nutrition.* 133, no. 11 (November 1, 2003): 3893S–3897.

Leiter, Lawrence A., Antonio Ceriello, Jaime A. Davidson, Markolf Hanefeld, Louis Monnier, David R. Owens, Naoko Tajima, and Jaakko Tuomilehto. "Postprandial glucose regulation: new data and new implications." *Clinical Therapeutics* 27 Suppl B (2005): S42–56.

Lessof, M.H. "Adverse reactions to food additives." *Journal of the Royal College of Physicians of London* 21, no. 4 (October 1987): 237–240.

——. "Food intolerance and allergy—a review." *The Quarterly Journal of Medicine* 52, no. 206 (1983): 111–119.

Lieberman, Shari. *Transitions Lifestyle System Glycemic Index Food Guide.* Unknown, 2006.

Lieberman, Shari, and James J. Gormley. *User's Guide to Detoxification. 1st ed.* Basic Health Publications, 2005.

Livesey, Geoffrey. "Low-glycaemic diets and health: implications for obesity." *The Proceedings of the Nutrition Society* 64, no. 1 (February 2005): 105–113.

Livesey, Geoffrey, Richard Taylor, Toine Hulshof, and John Howlett. "Glycemic response and health—a systematic review and meta-analysis: relations between dietary glycemic properties and health outcomes." *The American Journal of Clinical Nutrition* 87, no. 1 (January 2008): 258S–268S.

Logan, Alan C. "Neurobehavioral aspects of omega-3 fatty acids: possible mechanisms and therapeutic value in major depression." *Alternative Medicine Review: A Journal of Clinical Therapeutic* 8, no. 4 (November 2003): 410–425.

——. "Omega-3 fatty acids and major depression: A primer for the mental health professional." *Lipids in Health and Disease* 3 (n.d.): 25.

Ludwig, David S. "The glycemic index: physiological mechanisms relating to obesity, diabetes, and cardiovascular disease." *JAMA: The Journal of the American Medical Association* 287, no. 18 (May 8, 2002): 2414–2423.

Madrazo, Jose A., and Daniel P. Kelly. "The PPAR trio: regulators of myocardial energy metabolism in health and disease." *Journal of Molecular and Cellular Cardiology* 44, no. 6 (June 2008): 968–975.

Mainardi, Elsa, Alessandro Montanelli, Maria Dotti, Rosanna Nano, and Gianna Moscato. "Thyroid-related autoantibodies and celiac disease: a role for a gluten-free diet?." *Journal of Clinical Gastroenterology* 35, no. 3 (September 2002): 245–248.

Maintz, Laura, and Natalija Novak. "Histamine and histamine intolerance." *The American Journal of Clinical Nutrition* 85, no. 5 (May 2007): 1185–1196.

McGough, Norma, and John H. Cummings. "Coeliac disease: a diverse clinical syndrome caused by intolerance of wheat, barley and rye." *Proceedings of the Nutrition Society* 64, no. 04 (2005): 434–450.

Millward, D.J. "The nutritional value of plant-based diets in relation to human amino acid and protein requirements." *The Proceedings of the Nutrition Society* 58, no. 2 (May 1999): 249–260.

Millward, D. Joe, Donald K. Layman, Daniel Tome, and Gertjan Schaafsma. "Protein quality assessment: impact of expanding understanding of protein and amino acid needs for optimal health." *The American Journal of Clinical Nutrition* 87, no. 5 (May 1, 2008): 1576S–1581.

Minor, Robin K., Joanne S. Allard, Caitlin M. Younts, Theresa M. Ward, and Rafael de Cabo. "Dietary interventions to extend life span and health span based on calorie restriction." *The Journals of Gerontology. Series A, Biological Sciences and Medical Sciences* 65, no. 7 (July 2010): 695–703.

Nakatani, N. "Phenolic antioxidants from herbs and spices." *Bio-

Factors (Oxford, England) 13, no. 1 (2000): 141–146.

NutriBase. *The NutriBase Complete Book of Food Counts. 2nd ed.* Avery Trade, 2001.

O'Keefe, James H., and Loren Cordain. "Cardiovascular disease resulting from a diet and lifestyle at odds with our paleolithic genome: how to become a 21st-century hunter-gatherer." *Mayo Clinic Proceedings* 79, no. 1 (January 1, 2004): 101–108.

Ortolani, C, and E. Pastorello. "Food allergies and food intolerances." *Best Practice & Research Clinical Gastroenterology* 20, no. 3 (2006): 467–483.

Pace-Asciak, Cecil R., Susan Hahn, Eleftherios P. Diamandis, George Soleas, and David M. Goldberg. "The red wine phenolics trans-resveratrol and quercetin block human platelet aggregation and eicosanoid synthesis: implications for protection against coronary heart disease." *Clinica Chimica Acta* 235, no. 2 (March 31, 1995): 207–219.

Parker, S.L, G.L. Sussman, and M. Krondl. "Dietary aspects of adverse reactions to foods in adults." *CMAJ: Canadian Medical Association Journal = Journal De l'Association Medicale Canadienne* 139, no. 8 (October 15, 1988): 711–718.

Petersburg, Gregory W. "Living Younger Preventive-Aging Medicine Business System", 2007

Randhawa, Shahid, and Sami L. Bahna. "Hypersensitivity reactions to food additives." *Current Opinion in Allergy and Clinical Immunology* 9, no. 3 (June 2009): 278–283.

Salmerón, J., A. Ascherio, E.B. Rimm, G.A. Colditz, D. Spiegelman, D.J. Jenkins, M.J. Stampfer, A.L. Wing, and W.C. Willett. "Dietary fiber, glycemic load, and risk of NIDDM in men." *Diabetes Care* 20, no. 4 (April 1997): 545–550.

Sandberg, Ann-Sofie. "Bioavailability of minerals in legumes." *The British Journal of Nutrition* 88 Suppl 3 (December 2002): S281–285.

Sansoni, P., R. Vescovini, F. Fagnoni, C. Biasini, F. Zanni, L. Zanlari, A. Telera, et al. "The immune system in extreme longevity." *Experimental Gerontology* 43, no. 2 (February 2008): 61–65.

Savaiano, D.A., and C. Kotz. "Recent advances in the management of lactose intolerance." *ASDC Journal of Dentistry for Children* 56, no. 3 (June 1989): 228–233.

Semeniuk, J., and M. Kaczmarski. "Gastroesophageal reflux (GER) in children and adolescents with regard to food intolerance." *Advances in Medical Sciences* 51 (2006): 321–326.

Shaukat, Aasma, Michael D. Levitt, Brent C. Taylor, Roderick MacDonald, Tatyana A. Shamliyan, Robert L. Kane, and Timothy J. Wilt. "Systematic review: effective management strategies for lactose intolerance." *Annals of Internal Medicine* 152, no. 12 (June 15, 2010): 797–803.

Simopoulos, A.P. "Human requirement for N-3 polyunsaturated fatty acids." *Poultry Science* 79, no. 7 (July 2000): 961–970.

———. "Omega-3 fatty acids in health and disease and in growth and development." *The American Journal of Clinical Nutrition* 54, no. 3 (September 1991): 438–463.

Simopoulos, Artemis P. "The importance of the omega-6/omega-3 fatty acid ratio in cardiovascular disease and other chronic diseases." *Experimental Biology and Medicine (Maywood, N.J.)* 233, no. 6 (June 2008): 674–688.

Solomon, C.G., and J.E. Manson. "Obesity and mortality: a review of the epidemiologic data." *The American Journal of Clinical Nutrition* 66, no. 4 (October 1997): 1044S–1050S.

Specker, B.L. "Nutritional concerns of lactating women consuming vegetarian diets." *The American Journal of Clinical Nutrition* 59, no. 5 (May 1994): 1182S–1186S.

Tapsell, Linda C., Ian Hemphill, Lynne Cobiac, Craig S. Patch, David R. Sullivan, Michael Fenech, Steven Roodenrys, et al. "Health benefits of herbs and spices: the past, the present, the future." *The Medical Journal of Australia* 185, no. 4 (August 21, 2006): S4–24.

Temelkova-Kurktschiev, T.S, C. Koehler, E. Henkel, W. Leonhardt, K. Fuecker, and M. Hanefeld. "Postchallenge plasma glucose and glycemic spikes are more strongly associated with atherosclerosis than fasting glucose or HbA1c level." *Diabetes Care* 23, no. 12 (December 2000): 1830–1834.

Thomas, D.E., E.J. Elliott, and L. Baur. "Low glycaemic index or low glycaemic load diets for overweight and obesity." *Cochrane Database of Systematic Reviews (Online)*, no. 3 (2007): CD005105.

Transitions Lifestyle System Easy-to-Use Glycemic Index Food Guide. Square One Publishers, 2006.

Wantke, F., M. Götz, and R. Jarisch. "Histamine-free diet: treatment of choice for histamine-induced food intolerance and supporting treatment for chronic headaches." *Clinical and Experimental Allergy: Journal of the British Society for Allergy and Clinical Immunology* 23, no. 12 (December 1993): 982–985.

Westerterp-Plantenga, M.S., A. Nieuwenhuizen, D. Tomé, S. Soenen, and K.R. Westerterp. "Dietary protein, weight loss, and weight maintenance." *Annual Review of Nutrition* 29 (2009): 21–41.

Willcox, D. Craig, Bradley J. Willcox, Hidemi Todoriki, and Makoto Suzuki. "The Okinawan diet: health implications of a low-calorie, nutrient-dense, antioxidant-rich dietary pattern low in glycemic load." *Journal of the American College of Nutrition* 28 Suppl (August 2009): 500S–516S.

Worm, M., W. Vieth, I. Ehlers, W. Sterry, and T. Zuberbier. "Increased leukotriene production by food additives in patients with atopic dermatitis and proven food intolerance." *Clinical & Experimental Allergy* 31, no. 2 (2, 2001): 265–273.

Ye, Jianping, and Jeffrey N. Keller. "Regulation of energy metabolism by inflammation: a feedback response in obesity and calorie restriction." *Aging* 2, no. 6 (June 2010): 361–368.

Young, E., S. Patel, M. Stoneham, R. Rona, and J.D. Wilkinson. "The prevalence of reaction to food additives in a survey population." *Journal of the Royal College of Physicians of*

London 21, no. 4 (October 1987): 241–247.

Young, V.R., and P.L. Pellett. "Plant proteins in relation to human protein and amino acid nutrition." *The American Journal of Clinical Nutrition* 59, no. 5 (May 1994): 1203S–1212S.

——. "Protein intake and requirements with reference to diet and health." *The American Journal of Clinical Nutrition* 45, no. 5 (May 1987): 1323–1343.

Zanovec, Michael, Carol E. O'Neil, Debra R. Keast, Victor L. Fulgoni, and Theresa A. Nicklas. "Lean beef contributes significant amounts of key nutrients to the diets of US adults: National Health and Nutrition Examination Survey 1999–2004." *Nutrition Research (New York, N.Y.)* 30, no. 6 (June 2010): 375–381.

Zheng, W., and S.Y. Wang. "Antioxidant activity and phenolic compounds in selected herbs." *Journal of Agricultural and Food Chemistry* 49, no. 11 (November 2001): 5165–5170.

Chapter 3: Supplement Savvy

Ames, Bruce N. "Low micronutrient intake may accelerate the degenerative diseases of aging through allocation of scarce micronutrients by triage." *Proceedings of the National Academy of Sciences of the United States of America* 103, no. 47 (November 21, 2006): 17589–17594.

Anderson, J.J.B., C.M. Suchindran, and K.J. Roggenkamp. "Micronutrient intakes in two US populations of older adults: lipid research clinics program prevalence study findings." *The Journal of Nutrition, Health & Aging* 13, no. 7 (August 2009): 595–600.

Anderson, James W., Pat Baird, Richard H. Davis, Stefanie Ferreri, Mary Knudtson, Ashraf Koraym, Valerie Waters, and Christine L Williams. "Health benefits of dietary fiber." *Nutrition Reviews* 67, no. 4 (April 2009): 188–205.

Balch, CNC, Phyllis A. *Prescription for Nutritional Healing: A Practical A-to-Z Reference to Drug-Free Remedies Using Vitamins, Minerals, Herbs & Food Supplements. 5th ed.* Avery Trade, 2010.

Barabino, Stefano, Maurizio Rolando, Paola Camicione, Giambattista Ravera, Sabrina Zanardi, Sebastiano Giuffrida, and Giovanni Calabria. "Systemic linoleic and gamma-linolenic acid therapy in dry eye syndrome with an inflammatory component." *Cornea* 22, no. 2 (March 2003): 97–101.

Chatfield, S.M., C. Brand, P.R. Ebeling, and D.M. Russell. "Vitamin D deficiency in general medical inpatients in summer and winter." *Internal Medicine Journal* 37, no. 6 (June 2007): 377–382.

Cherniack, E. Paul, Silvina Levis, and Bruce R. Troen. "Hypovitaminosis D: a widespread epidemic." *Geriatrics* 63, no. 4 (April 2008): 24–30.

Craig, Winston J. "Health effects of vegan diets." *The American Journal of Clinical Nutrition* 89, no. 5 (May 2009): 1627S–1633S.

Dangour, Alan D., Sakhi K. Dodhia, Arabella Hayter, Elizabeth Allen, Karen Lock, and Ricardo Uauy. "Nutritional quality of organic foods: a systematic review." *The American Journal of Clinical Nutrition* 90, no. 3 (September 2009): 680–685.

Davis, Donald R., Melvin D. Epp, and Hugh D. Riordan. "Changes in USDA food composition data for 43 garden crops, 1950 to 1999." *Journal of the American College of Nutrition* 23, no. 6 (December 1, 2004): 669–682.

"Dietary Guidelines for Americans 2005." USDHHS USDA, n.d.

"Dietary Supplement Fact Sheet: Calciium." NIH: ODS, n.d.

Dixon, T., P. Mitchell, T. Beringer, S. Gallacher, C. Moniz, S. Patel, G. Pearson, and P. Ryan. "An overview of the prevalence of 25-hydroxy-vitamin D inadequacy amongst elderly patients with or without fragility fracture in the United Kingdom." *Current Medical Research and Opinion* 22, no. 2 (February 2006): 405–415.

Druss, Benjamin G., Steven C. Marcus, Mark Olfson, Terri Tanielian, and Harold Alan Pincus. "Trends in care by nonphysician clinicians in the United States." *New England Journal of Medicine* 348, no. 2 (January 9, 2003): 130–137.

Eades, Mary Dan. *The Doctor's Complete Guide to Vitamins and Minerals. Revised.* Dell, 2000.

Eisenberg, David M., Roger B. Davis, Susan L. Ettner, Scott Appel, Sonja Wilkey, Maria Van Rompay, and Ronald C. Kessler. "Trends in alternative medicine use in the United States, 1990—1997: results of a follow-up national survey." *JAMA: The Journal of the American Medical Association* 280, no. 18 (November 11, 1998): 1569–1575.

Hendler Ph.D, M.D, Sheldon; and David Rorvik. *PDR for Nutritional Supplements. Second Edition.* PDR Network, 2008.

Kaur, Narinder, and Anil K. Gupta. "Applications of inulin and oligofructose in health and nutrition." *Journal of Biosciences* 27, no. 7 (December 2002): 703–714.

Kelly, G.S. "Folates: supplemental forms and therapeutic applications." *Alternative Medicine Review: A Journal of Clinical Therapeutic* 3, no. 3 (June 1998): 208–220.

LaValle, James B., and Stacy Lundin Yale. *Cracking the Metabolic Code. 1st ed.* Basic Health Publications, Inc., 2003.

Long, Amanda N., Mario M. Ray, Deepak Nandikanti, Benjamin Bowman, Amna Khan, Kimberly Lamar, Tom Hughes, Patricia Adams-Graves, and Beverly Williams-Cleaves. "Prevalence of 25-hydroxyvitamin D deficiency in an urban general internal medicine academic practice." *Tennessee Medicine: Journal of the Tennessee Medical Association* 103, no. 7 (August 2010): 51–52, 57.

Lucock, Mark, and Zoe Yates. "Folic acid fortification: a double-edged sword." *Current Opinion in Clinical Nutrition and Metabolic Care* 12, no. 6 (November 2009): 555–564.

Macrì, Angelo, Sebastiano Giuffrida, Valentina Amico, Michele Iester, and Carlo Enrico Traverso. "Effect of linoleic acid and gamma-linolenic acid on tear production, tear clearance and on the ocular surface after photorefractive keratectomy." *Graefe's Archive for Clinical and Experimental Ophthalmology = Albrecht Von Graefes Archiv Für Klinische Und Experimentelle Ophthalmologie* 241, no. 7 (July 2003):

561–566.

"Magnesium," n.d. ods.od.nih.gov/factsheets/magnesium.asp#en28.

"Magnesium fact sheet ODS NIH." National Institutes of Health, Office of Dietary Supplements, n.d.

Mansoor, Shireen, Aysha Habib, Farooq Ghani, Zafar Fatmi, Salma Badruddin, Sarwat Mansoor, Imran Siddiqui, and Abdul Jabbar. "Prevalence and significance of vitamin D deficiency and insufficiency among apparently healthy adults." *Clinical Biochemistry* (September 25, 2010). www.ncbi.nlm.nih.gov/pubmed/20875809.

McKinley, M.C. "Nutritional aspects and possible pathological mechanisms of hyperhomocysteinaemia: an independent risk factor for vascular disease." *The Proceedings of the Nutrition Society* 59, no. 2 (May 2000): 221–237.

Messina, V., and A.R. Mangels. "Considerations in planning vegan diets: children." *Journal of the American Dietetic Association* 101, no. 6 (June 2001): 661–669.

Nielsen, Forrest H. "Magnesium, inflammation, and obesity in chronic disease." *Nutrition Reviews* 68, no. 6 (June 2010): 333–340.

Park, Sohyun, and Mary Ann Johnson. "Living in low-latitude regions in the United States does not prevent poor vitamin D status." *Nutrition Reviews* 63, no. 6 (June 2005): 203–209.

PDR for Herbal Medicines. 4th Edition. Thomson Reuters, 2007.

Petersburg, Gregory W. "Living Younger Preventive-Aging Medicine Business System", 2007

Pinheiro, Manuel Neuzimar, Procópio Miguel dos Santos, Regina Cândido Ribeiro dos Santos, Jeison de Nadai Barros, Luiz Fernando Passos, and José Cardoso Neto. "[Oral flaxseed oil (Linum usitatissimum) in the treatment for dry-eye Sjögren's syndrome patients]." *Arquivos Brasileiros De Oftalmologia* 70, no. 4 (August 2007): 649–655.

Säemann, Marcus D., Georg A. Böhmig, and Gerhard J. Zlabinger. "Short-chain fatty acids: bacterial mediators of a balanced host-microbial relationship in the human gut." *Wiener Klinische Wochenschrift* 114, no. 8 (May 15, 2002): 289–300.

Segala, Melanie. *Disease Prevention & Treatment. 4th ed.* Life Extension Publications Inc., 2003.

Smith, A. David, Stephen M. Smith, Celeste A. de Jager, Philippa Whitbread, Carole Johnston, Grzegorz Agacinski, Abderrahim Oulhaj, Kevin M. Bradley, Robin Jacoby, and Helga Refsum. "Homocysteine-lowering by B vitamins slows the rate of accelerated brain atrophy in mild cognitive impairment: a randomized controlled trial." *PLoS ONE* 5, no. 9 (2010): e12244.

Smith, M.D., Pamela Wartian. *What You Must Know About Vitamins, Minerals, Herbs, & More: Choosing the Nutrients That Are Right for You. 1st ed.* Square One Publishers, 2008.

Stacewicz-Sapuntzakis, M., P.E. Bowen, E.A. Hussain, B.I. Damayanti-Wood, and N.R. Farnsworth. "Chemical composition and potential health effects of prunes: a functional food?." *Critical Reviews in Food Science and Nutrition* 41, no. 4 (May 2001): 251–286.

Stanger, O. "Physiology of folic acid in health and disease." *Current Drug Metabolism* 3, no. 2 (April 2002): 211–223.

Stechschulte, Sarah A., Robert S. Kirsner, and Daniel G. Federman. "Vitamin D: bone and beyond, rationale and recommendations for supplementation." *The American Journal of Medicine* 122, no. 9 (September 2009): 793–802.

Strain, J.J., L. Dowey, M. Ward, K. Pentieva, and H. McNulty. "B-vitamins, homocysteine metabolism and CVD." *The Proceedings of the Nutrition Society* 63, no. 4 (November 2004): 597–603.

"Vitamin A fact sheet NIH ODS," n.d.

Wilson, C.P., H. McNulty, J.M. Scott, J.J. Strain, and M. Ward. "Postgraduate symposium: the MTHFR C677T polymorphism, B-vitamins and blood pressure." *The Proceedings of the Nutrition Society* 69, no. 1 (February 2010): 156–165.

Worthington, V. "Effect of agricultural methods on nutritional quality: a comparison of organic with conventional crops." *Alternative Therapies in Health and Medicine* 4, no. 1 (January 1998): 58–69.

Chapter 4: Be FIT–BE SaFE

American College of Sports Medicine. *ACSM's Guidelines for Exercise Testing and Prescription. Eighth.* Lippincott Williams & Wilkins, 2009.

"American College of Sports Medicine position stand. Progression models in resistance training for healthy adults." *Medicine and Science in Sports and Exercise* 41, no. 3 (March 2009): 687–708.

Anderson, Bob, and Jean Anderson. *Stretching: 20th anniversary.* Shelter Publications, Inc., 2000.

Baker, Laura D., Laura L. Frank, Karen Foster-Schubert, Pattie S. Green, Charles W. Wilkinson, Anne McTiernan, Stephen R. Plymate, et al. "Effects of aerobic exercise on mild cognitive impairment: a controlled trial." *Archives of Neurology* 67, no. 1 (January 2010): 71–79.

Charro, M.A., M.S. Aoki, A.J. Coutts, R.C. Araújo, and R.F. Bacurau. "Hormonal, metabolic and perceptual responses to different resistance training systems." *The Journal of Sports Medicine and Physical Fitness* 50, no. 2 (June 2010): 229–234.

Delavier, Frederic. *Strength Training Anatomy. 3rd Edition.* Human Kinetics, 2010.

Forbes, G.B. "Longitudinal changes in adult fat-free mass: influence of body weight." *The American Journal of Clinical Nutrition* 70, no. 6 (December 1999): 1025–1031.

Fry, A.C., and C.A. Lohnes. "Acute testosterone and cortisol responses to high power resistance exercise." *Fiziologiia Cheloveka* 36, no. 4 (August 2010): 102–106.

Jonas, Steven, and Edward M. Phillips. *ACSM's Exercise is Medicine: A Clinician's Guide to Exercise Prescription. 1st ed.* Lippincott Williams & Wilkins, 2009.

Kraemer, W.J., R.S. Staron, F.C. Hagerman, R.S. Hikida, A.C. Fry, S.E. Gordon, B.C. Nindl, et al. "The effects of short-term resistance training on endocrine function in men and women." *European Journal of Applied Physiology and Occupational Physiology* 78, no. 1 (June 1998): 69–76.

Lucidi, Paola, Paolo Rossetti, Francesca Porcellati, Simone Pampanelli, Paola Candeloro, Anna Marinelli Andreoli, Gabriele Perriello, Geremia B. Bolli, and Carmine G. Fanelli. "Mechanisms of insulin resistance after insulin-induced hypoglycemia in humans: the role of lipolysis." *Diabetes* 59, no. 6 (June 2010): 1349–1357.

McArdle, William D., Frank I. Katch, and Victor L. Katch. *Exercise Physiology, North American Edition: Nutrition, Energy, and Human Performance Point. Seventh.* Lippincott Williams & Wilkins, 2009.

National Strength and Conditioning Association. *Essentials of Strength Training and Conditioning. 3rd Edition.* Human Kinetics, 2008.

Petersburg, Gregory W. "Living Younger Preventive-Aging Medicine Business System", 2007

Rahimi, Rahman, Mohammad Qaderi, Hassan Faraji, and Saeed S. Boroujerdi. "Effects of very short rest periods on hormonal responses to resistance exercise in men." *Journal of Strength and Conditioning Research/National Strength & Conditioning Association* 24, no. 7 (July 2010): 1851–1859.

Roemmich, J.N., and A.D. Rogol. "Exercise and growth hormone: does one affect the other?" *The Journal of Pediatrics* 131, no. 1 (July 1997): S75–80.

Salles, Belmiro Freitas de, Roberto Simão, Fabrício Miranda, Jefferson da Silva Novaes, Adriana Lemos, and Jeffrey M. Willardson. "Rest interval between sets in strength training." *Sports Medicine (Auckland, N.Z.)* 39, no. 9 (2009): 765–777.

Shephard, R.J., and P.N. Shek. "Exercise, aging and immune function." *International Journal of Sports Medicine* 16, no. 1

(January 1995): 1–6.

Shinkai, S., M. Konishi, and R.J. Shephard. "Aging and immune response to exercise." *Canadian Journal of Physiology and Pharmacology* 76, no. 5 (May 1998): 562–572.

Stiegler, Petra, and Adam Cunliffe. "The role of diet and exercise for the maintenance of fat-free mass and resting metabolic rate during weight loss." *Sports Medicine (Auckland, N.Z.)* 36, no. 3 (2006): 239–262.

Stokes, Keith. "Growth hormone responses to sub-maximal and sprint exercise." *Growth Hormone & IGF Research: Official Journal of the Growth Hormone Research Society and the International IGF Research Society* 13, no. 5 (October 2003): 225–238.

Venjatraman, J. T., and G. Fernandes. "Exercise, immunity and aging." *Aging (Milan, Italy)* 9, no. 1 (April 1997): 42–56.

Weltman, A., L. Wideman, J.Y. Weltman, and J.D. Veldhuis. "Neuroendocrine control of GH release during acute aerobic exercise." *Journal of Endocrinological Investigation* 26, no. 9 (September 2003): 843–850.

Wideman, Laurie, Judy Y. Weltman, Mark L. Hartman, Johannes D. Veldhuis, and Arthur Weltman. "Growth hormone release during acute and chronic aerobic and resistance exercise: recent findings." *Sports Medicine (Auckland, N.Z.)* 32, no. 15 (2002): 987–1004.

Chapter 5: Hormone Harmony

Adam-Perrot, A., P. Clifton, and F. Brouns. "Low-carbohydrate diets: nutritional and physiological aspects." *Obesity Reviews: An Official Journal of the International Association for the Study of Obesity* 7, no. 1 (February 2006): 49–58.

Anagnostis, Panagiotis, Vasilios G. Athyros, Konstantinos Tziomalos, Asterios Karagiannis, and Dimitri P. Mikhailidis. "Clinical review: the pathogenetic role of cortisol in the metabolic syndrome: a hypothesis." *The Journal of Clinical Endocrinology and Metabolism* 94, no. 8 (August

2009): 2692–2701.

Cadore, Eduardo Lusa, Francisco Luiz Rodrigues Lhullier, Michel Arias Brentano, Eduardo Marczwski da Silva, Melissa Bueno Ambrosini, Rafael Spinelli, Rodrigo Ferrari Silva, and Luiz Fernando Martins Kruel. "Hormonal responses to resistance exercise in long-term trained and untrained middle-aged men." *Journal of Strength and Conditioning Research / National Strength & Conditioning Association* 22, no. 5 (September 2008): 1617–1624.

Casarez, Eli V., Marya E. Dunlap-Brown, Mark R. Conaway, and George P. Amorino. "Radiosensitization and modulation of p44/42 mitogen-activated protein kinase by 2-methoxyestradiol in prostate cancer models." *Cancer Research* 67, no. 17 (2007): 8316–8324.

Cree, Melanie G., Douglas Paddon-Jones, Bradley R. Newcomer, Ola Ronsen, Asle Aarsland, Robert R. Wolfe, and Arny Ferrando. "Twenty-eight-day bed rest with hypercortisolemia induces peripheral insulin resistance and increases intramuscular triglycerides." *Metabolism: Clinical and Experimental* 59, no. 5 (May 2010): 703–710.

Die, Margaret Diana van, Kerry M. Bone, Henry G. Burger, John E. Reece, and Helena J. Teede. "Effects of a combination of Hypericum perforatum and Vitex agnus-castus on PMS-like symptoms in late-perimenopausal women: findings from a subpopulation analysis." *Journal of Alternative and Complementary Medicine (New York, N.Y.)* 15, no. 9 (September 2009): 1045–1048.

Die, Margaret Diana van, Henry G. Burger, Helena J. Teede, and Kerry M. Bone. "Vitex agnus-castus (chaste-tree/berry) in the treatment of menopause-related complaints." *Journal of Alternative and Complementary Medicine (New York, N.Y.)* 15, no. 8 (August 2009): 853–862.

Geller, Stacie E., and Laura Studee. "Botanical and dietary supplements for menopausal symptoms: what works, what does not." *Journal of Women's Health (2002)* 14, no. 7 (September 2005): 634–649.

Grieb, Paweł, Barbara Kłapcińska, Ewelina Smol, Tomasz Pilis, Wiesław Pilis, Ewa Sadowska-Krepa, Andrzej Sobczak, et al. "Long-term consumption of a carbohydrate-restricted diet does not induce deleterious metabolic effects." *Nutrition Research (New York, N.Y.)* 28, no. 12 (December 2008): 825–833.

Heger, Marianne, Boris M. Ventskovskiy, Irina Borzenko, Kyra C. Kneis, Reinhard Rettenberger, Marietta Kaszkin-Bettag, and Peter W. Heger. "Efficacy and safety of a special extract of Rheum rhaponticum (ERr 731) in perimenopausal women with climacteric complaints: a 12-week randomized, double-blind, placebo-controlled trial." *Menopause (New York, N.Y.)* 13, no. 5 (October 2006): 744–759.

Jeppesen, Jørgen, Tine W. Hansen, Michael H. Olsen, Susanne Rasmussen, Hans Ibsen, Christian Torp-Pedersen, Per R. Hildebrandt, and Sten Madsbad. "C-reactive protein, insulin resistance and risk of cardiovascular disease: a population-based study." *European Journal of Cardiovascular Prevention and Rehabilitation: Official Journal of the European Society of Cardiology, Working Groups on Epidemiology & Prevention and Cardiac Rehabilitation and Exercise Physiology* 15, no. 5 (October 2008): 594–598.

Jeppesen, Jørgen, Tine W. Hansen, Susanne Rasmussen, Hans Ibsen, Christian Torp-Pedersen, and Sten Madsbad. "Insulin resistance, the metabolic syndrome, and risk of incident cardiovascular disease: a population-based study." *Journal of the American College of Cardiology* 49, no. 21 (May 29, 2007): 2112–2119.

Kamath, Kathy, Tatiana Okouneva, Gary Larson, Dulal Panda, Leslie Wilson, and Mary Ann Jordan. "2-Methoxyestradiol suppresses microtubule dynamics and arrests mitosis without depolymerizing microtubules." *Molecular Cancer Therapeutics* 5, no. 9 (2006): 2225–2233.

Kanadys, Wiesław Maciej, Bozena Leszczyńska-Gorzelak, and Jan Oleszczuk. "[Efficacy and safety of Black cohosh (Actaea/ Cimicifuga racemosa) in the treatment of vasomotor symptoms—review of clinical trials]." *Ginekologia Polska* 79, no. 4 (April 2008): 287–296.

Kaszkin-Bettag, Marietta, Sabine Beck, Andy Richardson, Peter W. Heger, and André-Michael Beer. "Efficacy of the special extract ERr 731 from rhapontic rhubarb for menopausal complaints: a 6-month open observational study." *Alternative Therapies in Health and Medicine* 14, no. 6 (December 2008): 32–38.

Kronenberg, Fredi, and Adriane Fugh-Berman. "Complementary and alternative medicine for menopausal symptoms: a review of randomized, controlled trials." *Annals of Internal Medicine* 137, no. 10 (November 19, 2002): 805–813.

LaVallee, Theresa M., Xiaoguo H. Zhan, Chris J. Herbstritt, Emily C. Kough, Shawn J. Green, and Victor S. Pribluda. "2-methoxyestradiol inhibits proliferation and induces apoptosis independently of estrogen receptors α and β." *Cancer Research* 62, no. 13 (July 1, 2002): 3691–3697.

Lewis, Michael I., Mario Fournier, Thomas W. Storer, Shalender Bhasin, Janos Porszasz, Song-Guang Ren, Xiaoyu Da, and Richard Casaburi. "Skeletal muscle adaptations to testosterone and resistance training in men with COPD." *Journal of Applied Physiology* 103, no. 4 (October 1, 2007): 1299–1310.

Loch, E.G., H. Selle, and N. Boblitz. "Treatment of premenstrual syndrome with a phytopharmaceutical formulation containing Vitex agnus castus." *Journal of Women's Health & Gender-Based Medicine* 9, no. 3 (April 2000): 315–320.

Lovallo, William R., Noha H. Farag, Andrea S. Vincent, Terrie L. Thomas, and Michael F. Wilson. "Cortisol responses to mental stress, exercise, and meals following caffeine intake in men and women." *Pharmacology Biochemistry and Behavior* 83, no. 3 (March 2006): 441–447.

Low Dog, Tieraona. "Menopause: a review of botanical dietary supplements." *The American Journal of Medicine* 118 Suppl 12B (December 19, 2005): 98–108.

Lucidi, Paola, Paolo Rossetti, Francesca Porcellati, Simone Pampanelli, Paola Candeloro, Anna Marinelli Andreoli, Gabriele Perriello, Geremia B Bolli, and Carmine G Fanelli. "Mechanisms of insulin resistance after insulin-induced hypoglycemia in humans: the role of lipolysis." *Diabetes* 59, no. 6 (June 2010): 1349–1357.

Mahady, Gail B., Daniel Fabricant, Lucas R. Chadwick, and Birgit Dietz. "Black cohosh: an alternative therapy for menopause?." *Nutrition in Clinical Care: An Official Publication of Tufts University* 5, no. 6 (December 2002): 283-289.

McCaulley, Grant O., Jeffrey M. McBride, Prue Cormie, Matthew B. Hudson, James L. Nuzzo, John C. Quindry, and N. Travis Triplett. "Acute hormonal and neuromuscular responses to hypertrophy, strength and power type resistance exercise." *European Journal of Applied Physiology* 105, no. 5 (12, 2008): 695–704.

Miquel, J., A. Ramirezbosca, J. Ramirezbosca, and J. Alperi. "Menopause: a review on the role of oxygen stress and favorable effects of dietary antioxidants." *Archives of Gerontology and Geriatrics* 42, no. 3 (5, 2006): 289–306.

Misra, Madhusmita, Miriam A. Bredella, Patrika Tsai, Nara Mendes, Karen K. Miller, and Anne Klibanski. "Lower growth hormone and higher cortisol are associated with greater visceral adiposity, intramyocellular lipids, and insulin resistance in overweight girls." *American Journal of Physiology - Endocrinology and Metabolism* 295, no. 2 (August 2008): E385–392.

Morton, Nicholas Michael. "Obesity and corticosteroids: 11beta-hydroxysteroid type 1 as a cause and therapeutic target in metabolic disease." *Molecular and Cellular Endocrinology* 316, no. 2 (March 25, 2010): 154–164.

Orsatti, F, E. Nahas, N. Maesta, J. Nahasneto, and R. Burini. "Plasma hormones, muscle mass and strength in resistance-trained postmenopausal women." *Maturitas* 59, no. 4 (4, 2008): 394–404.

Osmers, Ruediger, Michael Friede, Eckehard Liske, Joerg Schnitker, Johannes Freudenstein, and Hans-Heinrich Henneicke-von Zepelin. "Efficacy and safety of isopropanolic black cohosh extract for climacteric symptoms." *Obstetrics and Gynecology* 105, no. 5 (May 2005): 1074–1083.

Oxenkrug, Gregory F. "Metabolic syndrome, age-associated neuroendocrine disorders, and dysregulation of tryptophan-kynurenine metabolism." *Annals of the New York Academy of Sciences* 1199 (June 2010): 1–14.

Pasquali, R., V. Vicennati, A. Gambineri, and U. Pagotto. "Sex-dependent role of glucocorticoids and androgens in the pathophysiology of human obesity." *International Journal of Obesity (2005)* 32, no. 12 (December 2008): 1764–1779.

Pasquali, Renato, Valentina Vicennati, Mauro Cacciari, and Uberto Pagotto. "The hypothalamic-pituitary-adrenal axis activity in obesity and the metabolic syndrome." *Annals of the New York Academy of Sciences* 1083 (November 2006): 111–128.

Petersburg, Gregory W. "Living Younger Preventive-Aging Medicine Business System", 2007

Purnell, Jonathan Q., Steven E. Kahn, Mary H. Samuels, David Brandon, D. Lynn Loriaux, and John D. Brunzell. "Enhanced cortisol production rates, free cortisol, and 11beta-HSD-1 expression correlate with visceral fat and insulin resistance in men: effect of weight loss." *American Journal of Physiology - Endocrinology and Metabolism* 296, no. 2 (February 2009): E351–357.

Reynolds, Rebecca M., Javier Labad, Mark W.J. Strachan, Anke Braun, F. Gerry R. Fowkes, Amanda J. Lee, Brian M. Frier, Jonathan R. Seckl, Brian R. Walker, and Jackie F. Price. "Elevated fasting plasma cortisol is associated with ischemic heart disease and its risk factors in people with type 2 diabetes: the Edinburgh type 2 diabetes study." *The Journal of Clinical Endocrinology and Metabolism* 95, no. 4 (April 2010): 1602–1608.

Reynolds, Rebecca M., Mark W.J. Strachan, Javier Labad, Amanda J. Lee, Brian M. Frier, F. Gerald Fowkes, Rory Mitchell, et al. "Morning cortisol levels and cognitive abilities in people with type 2 diabetes: the Edinburgh type 2 diabetes study." *Diabetes Care* 33, no. 4 (April 2010): 714–720.

Rotem, Carmela, and Boris Kaplan. "Phyto-female complex for the relief of hot flushes, night sweats and quality of sleep: randomized, controlled, double-blind pilot study." *Gynecological Endocrinology: The Official Journal of the International Society of Gynecological Endocrinology* 23, no. 2 (February 2007): 117–122.

Rundek, Tatjana, Hannah Gardener, Qiang Xu, Ronald B. Goldberg, Clinton B. Wright, Bernadette Boden-Albala, Norbelina Disla, Myunghee C. Paik, Mitchell S.V. Elkind, and Ralph L. Sacco. "Insulin resistance and risk of ischemic stroke among nondiabetic individuals from the northern Manhattan study." *Archives of Neurology* 67, no. 10 (October 2010): 1195–1200.

Rutter, Martin K., James B. Meigs, Lisa M. Sullivan, Ralph B. D'Agostino, and Peter W. Wilson. "Insulin resistance, the metabolic syndrome, and incident cardiovascular events in the Framingham Offspring Study." *Diabetes* 54, no. 11 (November 2005): 3252–3257.

Ryan, A.S. "Insulin resistance with aging: effects of diet and exercise." *Sports Medicine (Auckland, N.Z.)* 30, no. 5 (November 2000): 327–346.

Sallinen, J., A. Pakarinen, M. Fogelholm, M. Alen, J. Volek, W. Kraemer, and K. Häkkinen. "Dietary intake, serum hormones, muscle mass and strength during strength training in 49-73-year-old men." *International Journal of Sports Medicine* 28, no. 12 (12, 2007): 1070–1076.

Schenk, Simon, Maziyar Saberi, and Jerrold M. Olefsky. "Insulin sensitivity: modulation by nutrients and inflammation." *Journal of Clinical Investigation* 118, no. 9 (9, 2008): 2992–3002.

Shang, Weirong, Ioanna Konidari, and David W. Schomberg. "2-Methoxyestradiol, an endogenous estradiol metabolite, differentially inhibits granulosa and endothelial cell mitosis: a potential follicular antiangiogenic regulator." *Biology of Reproduction* 65, no. 2 (2001): 622–627.

Smith, M.D., Pamela Wartian. *What You Must Know About Women's Hormones: Your Guide to Natural Hormone Treatents for PMS, Menopause, Osteoporosis, PCOS, and More. 1st ed.* Square One Publishers, 2009.

Walker, B.R. "Cortisol—cause and cure for metabolic syndrome?" *Diabetic Medicine: A Journal of the British Diabetic Association* 23, no. 12 (December 2006): 1281–1288.

Yarrow, Joshua F., Paul A. Borsa, Stephen E. Borst, Harry S. Sitren, Bruce R. Stevens, and Lesley J. White. "Early-phase neuroendocrine responses and strength adaptations following eccentric-enhanced resistance training." *Journal of Strength and Conditioning Research/National Strength & Conditioning Association* 22, no. 4 (July 2008): 1205–1214.

Chapter 6: Stress Less, Age Less

Benson, M.D., Herbert, and Miriam Z. Klipper. *The Relaxation Response. Exp Upd.* Harper Paperbacks, 2000.

Chiesa, Alberto, and Alessandro Serretti. "Mindfulness-based stress reduction for stress management in healthy people: a review and meta-analysis." *Journal of Alternative and Complementary Medicine (New York, N.Y.)* 15, no. 5 (May 2009): 593–600.

Chrousos, G.P. "The role of stress and the hypothalamic-pituitary-adrenal axis in the pathogenesis of the metabolic syndrome: neuro-endocrine and target tissue-related causes." *International Journal of Obesity and Related Metabolic Disorders: Journal of the International Association for the Study of Obesity* 24 Suppl 2 (June 2000): S50–55.

Epel, Elissa, Jennifer Daubenmier, Judith Tedlie Moskowitz, Susan Folkman, and Elizabeth Blackburn. "Can meditation slow rate of cellular aging? Cognitive stress, mindfulness, and telomeres." *Annals of the New York Academy of Sciences* 1172 (August 2009): 34–53.

Habib, K.E., P.W. Gold, and G.P. Chrousos. "Neuroendocrinology of stress." *Endocrinology and Metabolism Clinics of North America* 30, no. 3 (September 2001): 695–728; vii–viii.

Jain, Shamini, Shauna L. Shapiro, Summer Swanick, Scott C. Roesch, Paul J. Mills, Iris Bell, and Gary E.R. Schwartz. "A randomized controlled trial of mindfulness meditation versus relaxation training: effects on distress, positive states of mind, rumination, and distraction." *Annals of Behavioral Medicine: A Publication of the Society of Behavioral Medicine* 33, no. 1 (February 2007): 11–21.

Klink, J.J. van der, R.W. Blonk, A.H. Schene, and F.J. van Dijk. "The benefits of interventions for work-related stress." *American Journal of Public Health* 91, no. 2 (February 2001): 270–276.

Lehrer, PhD, Paul M., Robert L. Woolfolk, Phd, Wesley E. Sime, PhD, and David H. Barlow, PhD. *Principles and Practice of Stress Management. Third Edition.* The Guilford Press, 2008.

Lehrer, P.M., R. Carr, D. Sargunaraj, and R.L. Woolfolk. "Stress management techniques: are they all equivalent, or do they have specific effects?" *Biofeedback and Self-Regulation* 19, no. 4 (December 1994): 353–401.

Lovallo, William R., Noha H. Farag, Andrea S. Vincent, Terrie L. Thomas, and Michael F. Wilson. "Cortisol responses to mental stress, exercise, and meals following caffeine intake in men and women." *Pharmacology Biochemistry and Behavior* 83, no. 3 (March 2006): 441–447.

McMorris, Terry, Jon Swain, Marcus Smith, Jo Corbett, Simon Delves, Craig Sale, Roger C. Harris, and Julia Potter. "Heat stress, plasma concentrations of adrenaline, noradrenaline, 5-hydroxytryptamine and cortisol, mood state and cognitive performance." *International Journal of Psychophysiology* 61, no. 2 (August 2006): 204–215.

Murphy, L.R. "Stress management in work settings: a critical review of the health effects." *American Journal of Health Promotion: AJHP* 11, no. 2 (December 1996): 112–135.

Peavy, G., K. Lange, D. Salmon, T. Patterson, S. Goldman, A. Gamst, P. Mills, S. Khandrika, and D. Galasko. "The effects of prolonged stress and APOE genotype on memory and cortisol in older adults." *Biological Psychiatry* 62, no. 5 (9, 2007): 472–478.

Petersburg, Gregory W. "Living Younger Preventive-Aging Medicine Business System", 2007

Praissman, Sharon. "Mindfulness-based stress reduction: a literature review and clinician's guide." *Journal of the American Academy of Nurse Practitioners* 20, no. 4 (April 2008): 212–216.

Smeets, Tom, Henry Otgaar, Ingrid Candel, and Oliver T. Wolf. "True or false? Memory is differentially affected by stress-induced cortisol elevations and sympathetic activity at consolidation and retrieval." *Psychoneuroendocrinology* 33, no. 10 (November 2008): 1378–1386.

Spence, J.D., P.A. Barnett, W. Linden, V. Ramsden, and P. Taenzer. "Lifestyle modifications to prevent and control hypertension. 7. Recommendations on stress management. Canadian Hypertension Society, Canadian Coalition for High Blood Pressure Prevention and Control, Laboratory Centre for Disease Control at Health Canada, Heart and Stroke Foundation of Canada." *CMAJ: Canadian Medical Association Journal* 160, no. 9 (May 4, 1999): S46–S50.

Swaab, Dick F., Ai-Min Bao, and Paul J. Lucassen. "The stress system in the human brain in depression and neurodegeneration." *Ageing Research Reviews* 4, no. 2 (May 2005): 141–194.

Telles, S., and K.V. Naveen. "Yoga for rehabilitation: an overview." *Indian Journal of Medical Sciences* 51, no. 4 (April 1997): 123–127.

Telles, Shirley, Vaishali Gaur, and Acharya Balkrishna. "Effect of a yoga practice session and a yoga theory session on state anxiety." *Perceptual and Motor Skills* 109, no. 3 (December 2009): 924–930.

Chapter 7: Beyond the Basics

De la Fuente, M. "Effects of antioxidants on immune system ageing." *European Journal of Clinical Nutrition* 56 Suppl 3 (August 2002): S5–8.

Epel, Elissa S. "Psychological and metabolic stress: a recipe for accelerated cellular aging?" *Hormones (Athens, Greece)* 8, no. 1 (March 2009): 7–22.

Knight, J.A. "The biochemistry of aging." *Advances in Clinical Chemistry* 35 (2000): 1–62.

Lehninger, Albert, David L. Nelson, and Michael M. Cox. *Lehninger Principles of Biochemistry & eBook. Fifth Edition.* W.H. Freeman, 2008.

Ljubuncic, Predrag, and Abraham Z. Reznick. "The evolutionary theories of aging revisited—a mini-review." *Gerontology* 55, no. 2 (2009): 205–216.

Lord, Richard S. *Laboratory Evaluations for Integrative and Functional Medicine. 2nd ed.* Not Avail., 2008.

Marnett, L.J. "Chemistry and biology of DNA damage by malondialdehyde." *IARC Scientific Publications*, no. 150 (1999): 17–27.

——. "Lipid peroxidation-DNA damage by malondialdehyde." *Mutation Research* 424, no. 1 (March 8, 1999): 83–95.

Marnett, Lawrence J. "Oxy radicals, lipid peroxidation and DNA damage." *Toxicology* 181–182 (December 27, 2002): 219–222.

Miquel, J. "Nutrition and ageing." *Public Health Nutrition* 4, no. 6 (December 2001): 1385–1388.

Murray, Robert, Victor Rodwell, David Bender, Kathleen M. Botham, P. Anthony Weil, and Peter J. Kennelly. *Harper's Illustrated Biochemistry. 28th Edition.* McGraw-Hill Medical, 2009.

Oliveira, Barbara F., José Augusto Nogueira-Machado, and Míriam M. Chaves. "The role of oxidative stress in the aging process." *The Scientific World Journal* 10 (2010): 1121–1128.

Robert, L., J. Labat-Robert, and A.M. Robert. "Genetic, epigenetic and posttranslational mechanisms of aging." *Biogerontology* 11, no. 4 (August 2010): 387–399.

Squier, T.C. "Oxidative stress and protein aggregation during biological aging." *Experimental Gerontology* 36, no. 9 (September 2001): 1539–1550.

Chapter 8: Customized Care

Abbassy, A.S., M.M. Zeitoun, and M.H. Abouiwfa. "The state of vitamin B6 deficiency as measured by urinary xanthurenic acid." *Journal of Tropical Pediatrics* 5 (September 1959): 45–50.

Ames, Bruce N., Ilan Elson-Schwab, and Eli A. Silver. "High-dose vitamin therapy stimulates variant enzymes with decreased coenzyme binding affinity (increased Km): relevance to genetic disease and polymorphisms." *The American Journal of Clinical Nutrition* 75, no. 4 (April 1, 2002): 616–658.

Ashavaid, T.F., Seema P. Todur, and K.G. Nair. "Apolipoprotein E polymorphism and coronary heart disease." *The Journal of the Association of Physicians of India* 51 (August 2003): 784–788.

Baker, Sidney MacDonald, Peter Bennett, Jeffrey S. Bland, Leo Galland, Robert J. Hedaya, Mark Houston, Mark Hyman, Jay Lombard, Robert Rountree, and Alex Vasquez. *Textbook of Functional Medicine. Second.* 2005.

Barr, R. Graham, David M. Nathan, James B. Meigs, and Daniel E. Singer. "Tests of glycemia for the diagnosis of type 2 diabetes mellitus." *Annals of Internal Medicine* 137, no. 4 (August 20, 2002): 263–272.

Bland, Jeffrey S., Buck Levin, Linda Costarella, DeAnn Liska, Dan Lukaczer, Barbara Schiltz, Michael Schmidt, Robert Lerman, and David Jones. *Clinical Nutrition: A Functional Approach. 2nd Ed.* Institute of Functional Medicine, 2004.

Brewster, M.A. "Biomarkers of xenobiotic exposures." *Annals of Clinical and Laboratory Science* 18, no. 4 (August 1988):

306–317.

Chuang, David T., Jacinta L. Chuang, and R. Max Wynn. "Lessons from genetic disorders of branched-chain amino acid metabolism." *The Journal of Nutrition* 136, no. 1 (January 2006): 243S–9S.

Colayco, Danielle C., Fang Niu, Jeffrey S. McCombs, and T. Craig Cheetham. "Glycosylated hemoglobin and cardiovascular outcomes in type 2 diabetes: a nested case-control study." *Diabetes Care* (October 11, 2010). www.ncbi.nlm.nih.gov/pubmed/20937686.

Cortese, C., and C. Motti. "MTHFR gene polymorphism, homocysteine and cardiovascular disease." *Public Health Nutrition* 4, no. 2 (April 2001): 493–497.

Cullen, P. "Evidence that triglycerides are an independent coronary heart disease risk factor." *The American Journal of Cardiology* 86, no. 9 (November 1, 2000): 943–949.

Cziraky, Mark J., Karol E. Watson, and Robert L. Talbert. "Targeting low HDL-cholesterol to decrease residual cardiovascular risk in the managed care setting." *Journal of Managed Care Pharmacy: JMCP* 14, no. 8 (October 2008): S3–28; quiz S30–31.

Davignon, J., R.E. Gregg, and C.F. Sing. "Apolipoprotein E polymorphism and atherosclerosis." *Arteriosclerosis (Dallas, Tex.)* 8, no. 1 (February 1988): 1–21.

"Detection, evaluation and treatment of high blood cholesterol in adults ATP III final report." National Heart Lung and Blood Institute, n.d.

Goodwin, B.L., C.R. Ruthven, and M. Sandler. "Gut flora and the origin of some urinary aromatic phenolic compounds." *Biochemical Pharmacology* 47, no. 12 (June 15, 1994): 2294–2297.

Guldener, C. van, and C.D. Stehouwer. "Homocysteine-lowering treatment: an overview." *Expert Opinion on Pharmacotherapy* 2, no. 9 (September 2001): 1449–1460.

Hartweg, J., A.J. Farmer, R. Perera, R.R. Holman, and H.A.W.

Neil. "Meta-analysis of the effects of n-3 polyunsaturated fatty acids on lipoproteins and other emerging lipid cardiovascular risk markers in patients with type 2 diabetes." *Diabetologia* 50, no. 8 (August 2007): 1593–1602.

Hauser, Paul S., Vasanthy Narayanaswami, and Robert O. Ryan. "Apolipoprotein E: from lipid transport to neurobiology." *Progress in Lipid Research* (September 18, 2010). www.ncbi. nlm.nih.gov/pubmed/20854843.

He, J.A., X.H. Hu, Y.Y. Fan, J. Yang, Z.S. Zhang, C.W. Liu, D.H. Yang, et al. "Hyperhomocysteinaemia, low folate concentrations and methylene tetrahydrofolate reductase C677T mutation in acute mesenteric venous thrombosis." *European Journal of Vascular and Endovascular Surgery: The Official Journal of the European Society for Vascular Surgery* 39, no. 4 (April 2010): 508–513.

Hiraku, Y., M. Yamasaki, and S. Kawanishi. "Oxidative DNA damage induced by homogentisic acid, a tyrosine metabolite." *FEBS Letters* 432, no. 1 (July 31, 1998): 13–16.

Hooper, W. Craig, and Christine De Staercke. "Venous thromboembolism: implications for gene-based diagnosis and technology development." *Expert Review of Molecular Diagnostics* 2, no. 6 (November 2002): 576–586.

Huang, Yadong. "Mechanisms linking apolipoprotein E isoforms with cardiovascular and neurological diseases." *Current Opinion in Lipidology* 21, no. 4 (August 2010): 337–345.

Khandanpour, Nader, Gavin Willis, Felicity J. Meyer, Matthew P. Armon, Yoon K. Loke, Anthony J.A. Wright, Paul M. Finglas, and Barbara A. Jennings. "Peripheral arterial disease and methylenetetrahydrofolate reductase (MTHFR) C677T mutations: a case-control study and meta-analysis." *Journal of Vascular Surgery: Official Publication, the Society for Vascular Surgery [and] International Society for Cardiovascular Surgery, North American Chapter* 49, no. 3 (March 2009): 711–718.

Kim, Robert J., and Richard C. Becker. "Association between factor V Leiden, prothrombin G20210A, and methylenetetrahydrofolate reductase C677T mutations and events of the arterial circulatory system: a meta-analysis of published studies." *American Heart Journal* 146, no. 6 (December 2003): 948–957.

Lane, D.A., and P.J. Grant. "Role of hemostatic gene polymorphisms in venous and arterial thrombotic disease." *Blood* 95, no. 5 (March 1, 2000): 1517–1532.

Lehninger, Albert, David L. Nelson, and Michael M. Cox. *Lehninger Principles of Biochemistry & eBook. Fifth Edition.* W.H. Freeman, 2008.

Levin, Gregory, Bryan Kestenbaum, Yii-Der Ida Chen, David R. Jacobs, Bruce M. Psaty, Jerome I. Rotter, David S. Siscovick, and Ian H. de Boer. "Glucose, insulin, and incident hypertension in the multi-ethnic study of atherosclerosis." *American Journal of Epidemiology* (October 20, 2010). www.ncbi.nlm.nih.gov/pubmed/20961972.

Lipska, Kasia J., Nathalie De Rekeneire, Peter H. Van Ness, Karen C. Johnson, Alka Kanaya, Annemarie Koster, Elsa S. Strotmeyer, et al. "Identifying Dysglycemic States in Older Adults: Implications of the Emerging Use of Hemoglobin A1c." *The Journal of Clinical Endocrinology and Metabolism* (September 22, 2010). www.ncbi.nlm.nih.gov/pubmed/20861123.

Lord, Richard S. *Laboratory Evaluations for Integrative and Functional Medicine. 2nd ed.* Not avail., 2008.

Lord, Richard S., and J. Alexander Bralley. "Clinical applications of urinary organic acids. Part 1: Detoxification markers." *Alternative Medicine Review: A Journal of Clinical Therapeutic* 13, no. 3 (September 2008): 205–215.

———. "Clinical applications of urinary organic acids. Part 2. Dysbiosis markers." *Alternative Medicine Review: A Journal of Clinical Therapeutic* 13, no. 4 (December 2008): 292–306.

Luc, Gérald, Jean-Marie Bard, Dominique Arveiler, Jean Ferrieres, Alun Evans, Philippe Amouyel, Jean-Charles Fruchart, and Pierre Ducimetiere. "Lipoprotein (a) as a predictor of coronary heart disease: the PRIME study." *Atherosclerosis* 163, no. 2 (August 2002): 377–384.

Mahley, R.W., and S.C. Rall. "Apolipoprotein E: far more than a lipid transport protein." *Annual Review of Genomics and Human Genetics* 1 (2000): 507–537.

Miyaki, Koichi. "Genetic polymorphisms in homocysteine metabolism and response to folate intake: a comprehensive strategy to elucidate useful genetic information." *Journal of Epidemiology/Japan Epidemiological Association* 20, no. 4 (2010): 266–270.

Morgan, John M., Christina M. Carey, Anne Lincoff, and David M. Capuzzi. "The effects of niacin on lipoprotein subclass distribution." *Preventive Cardiology* 7, no. 4 (2004): 182–187; quiz 188.

Nakai, K., C. Itoh, K. Nakai, W. Habano, and D. Gurwitz. "Correlation between C677T MTHFR gene polymorphism, plasma homocysteine levels and the incidence of CAD." *American Journal of Cardiovascular Drugs: Drugs, Devices, and Other Interventions* 1, no. 5 (2001): 353–361.

"New triglyceride test could spot heart trouble earlier. Studies show non-fasting tests may be better predictors of cardiac events because they contain lipoprotein remnants not found in fasting tests." *Heart Advisor/The Cleveland Clinic* 10, no. 9 (September 2007): 5.

Noland, Robert C., Timothy R. Koves, Sarah E. Seiler, Helen Lum, Robert M. Lust, Olga Ilkayeva, Robert D. Stevens, Fausto G. Hegardt, and Deborah M. Muoio. "Carnitine insufficiency caused by aging and overnutrition compromises mitochondrial performance and metabolic control." *The Journal of Biological Chemistry* 284, no. 34 (August 21, 2009): 22840–22852.

Nordestgaard, Børge G., M. John Chapman, Kausik Ray, Jan Borén, Felicita Andreotti, Gerald F. Watts, Henry Ginsberg, et al. "Lipoprotein(a) as a cardiovascular risk factor: current status." *European Heart Journal* (October 21, 2010). www.ncbi.nlm.nih.gov/pubmed/20965889.

Ouguerram, K., C. Maugeais, J. Gardette, T. Magot, and M. Krempf. "Effect of n-3 fatty acids on metabolism of apoB100-containing lipoprotein in type 2 diabetic subjects." *The British Journal of Nutrition* 96, no. 1 (July 2006): 100–106.

Ozand, Pinar T., and Generoso G. Gascon. "Topical review article: organic acidurias: a review. Part 1." *Journal of Child Neurology* 6, no. 3 (July 1, 1991): 196 -219.

——. "Topical review article: organic acidurias: a review. Part 2." *Journal of Child Neurology* 6, no. 4 (October 1, 1991): 288–303.

Postiglione, A., G. Milan, A. Ruocco, G. Gallotta, G. Guiotto, and G. Di Minno. "Plasma folate, vitamin B(12), and total homocysteine and homozygosity for the C677T mutation of the 5,10-methylene tetrahydrofolate reductase gene in patients with Alzheimer's dementia. A case-control study." *Gerontology* 47, no. 6 (December 2001): 324–329.

Rizzo, M., and K. Berneis. "Who needs to care about small, dense low-density lipoproteins?" *International Journal of Clinical Practice* 61, no. 11 (November 2007): 1949–1956.

Rizzo, M., K. Berneis, E. Corrado, and S. Novo. "The significance of low-density-lipoproteins size in vascular diseases." *International Angiology: A Journal of the International Union of Angiology* 25, no. 1 (March 2006): 4–9.

Rizzo, M., G.B. Rini, and K. Berneis. "The clinical relevance of LDL size and subclasses modulation in patients with type-2 diabetes." *Experimental and Clinical Endocrinology & Diabetes: Official Journal, German Society of Endocrinology [and] German Diabetes Association* 115, no. 8 (September 2007): 477–482.

Ryan-Harshman, Milly, and Walid Aldoori. "Vitamin B12 and health." *Canadian Family Physician Médecin De Famille Canadien* 54, no. 4 (April 2008): 536–541.

Santangelo, Carmela, Rosaria Varì, Beatrice Scazzocchio, Roberta Di Benedetto, Carmela Filesi, and Roberta Masella. "Polyphenols, intracellular signalling and inflammation." *Annali dell'Istituto Superiore Di Sanità* 43, no. 4 (2007): 394–405.

Sarwar, Nadeem, Thor Aspelund, Gudny Eiriksdottir, Reeta Gobin, Sreenivasa Rao Kondapally Seshasai, Nita G Forouhi, Gunnar Sigurdsson, John Danesh, and Vilmundur Gudnason. "Markers of dysglycaemia and risk of coronary heart disease in people without diabetes: Reykjavik prospective study and systematic review." *PLoS Medicine* 7, no. 5 (2010): e1000278.

Sarwar, Nadeem, Naveed Sattar, Vilmundur Gudnason, and John Danesh. "Circulating concentrations of insulin markers and coronary heart disease: a quantitative review of 19 Western prospective studies." *European Heart Journal* 28, no. 20 (October 2007): 2491–2497.

Takahashi, Ryotaro, Akiko Imamura, Mari Yoshikane, Masayuki Suzuki, Ryuichiro Murakami, Xian Wu Cheng, Yasushi Numaguchi, Nobuo Ikeda, Toyoaki Murohara, and Kenji Okumura. "Very small low-density lipoprotein cholesterol level is a determinant of arterial stiffness in men with impaired glucose metabolism." *Journal of Atherosclerosis and Thrombosis* (September 8, 2010). www.ncbi.nlm.nih.gov/pubmed/20834193.

Thompson, A., and J. Danesh. "Associations between apolipoprotein B, apolipoprotein AI, the apolipoprotein B/AI ratio and coronary heart disease: a literature-based meta-analysis of prospective studies." *Journal of Internal Medicine* 259, no. 5 (May 2006): 481–492.

Tian, Li, and Mingde Fu. "The relationship between high density lipoprotein subclass profile and plasma lipids concentrations." *Lipids in Health and Disease* 9, no. 1 (October 17, 2010): 118.

Topic, Aleksandra, Vesna Spasojevic Kalimanovska, Aleksandra Zeljkovic, Jelena Vekic, and Zorana Jelic Ivanovic. "Gender-related effect of apo E polymorphism on lipoprotein particle sizes in the middle-aged subjects." *Clinical Biochemistry* 41, no. 6 (April 2008): 361–367.

Trabetti, Elisabetta. "Homocysteine, MTHFR gene polymorphisms, and cardio-cerebrovascular risk." *Journal of Applied Genetics* 49, no. 3 (2008): 267–282.

Wallace, D.C. "Mitochondrial genetics: a paradigm for aging and degenerative diseases?" *Science (New York, N.Y.)* 256, no. 5057 (May 1, 1992): 628–632.

———. "A mitochondrial paradigm for degenerative diseases and ageing." *Novartis Foundation Symposium* 235 (2001): 247–263; discussion 263–266.

Wallace, Douglas C. "A mitochondrial paradigm of metabolic and degenerative diseases, aging, and cancer: a dawn for evolutionary medicine." *Annual Review of Genetics* 39 (2005): 359–407.

Waugh, N., G. Scotland, P. McNamee, M. Gillett, A. Brennan, E. Goyder, R. Williams, and A. John. "Screening for type 2 diabetes: literature review and economic modelling." *Health Technology Assessment (Winchester, England)* 11, no. 17 (May 2007): iii–iv, ix–xi, 1–125.

Wooten, Joshua S., Kyle D. Biggerstaff, and Vic Ben-Ezra. "Responses of LDL and HDL particle size and distribution to omega-3 fatty acid supplementation and aerobic exercise." *Journal of Applied Physiology (Bethesda, Md.: 1985)* 107, no. 3 (September 2009): 794–800.

Wu, O., L. Robertson, S. Twaddle, G.D.O. Lowe, P. Clark, M. Greaves, I.D. Walker, et al. "Screening for thrombophilia in high-risk situations: systematic review and cost-effectiveness analysis. The Thrombosis: Risk and Economic Assessment of Thrombophilia Screening (TREATS) study." *Health Technology Assessment (Winchester, England)* 10, no. 11 (April 2006): 1–110.

Yoon, Joo-Heon, and Seung Joon Baek. "Molecular targets of dietary polyphenols with anti-inflammatory properties." *Yonsei Medical Journal* 46, no. 5 (October 31, 2005): 585–596.

Zee, Robert Y.L., Robert J. Glynn, Suzanne Cheng, Lori Steiner, Lynda Rose, and Paul M. Ridker. "An evaluation of candidate genes of inflammation and thrombosis in relation to the risk of venous thromboembolism: The Women's Genome Health Study." *Circulation. Cardiovascular Genetics* 2, no. 1 (February 2009): 57–62.

Appendices

American College of Sports Medicine. *ACSM's Health-Related Physical Fitness Assessment Manual. Third.* Lippincott Williams & Wilkins, 2009.

"ACSM physical activity guidelines," n.d. www.acsm.org/AM/Template.cfm?Section=Home_Page&TEMPLATE=CM/HTMLDisplay.cfm&CONTENTID=7764.

"Aging and Glycation." *Life Extension Magazine*, April 2008.

Anderson, Bob. *Stretching. Twenty-seventh.* Shelter Publications, Incorporated, 1980.

"Classification of overweight and obesity by BMI, waist circumference and associated disease risk." National Heart Lung and Blood Institute, n.d.

"A comprehensive guide to preventive blood testing." *Life Extension Magazine*, May 2004.

Danesh, J., R. Collins, P. Appleby, and R. Peto. "Association of fibrinogen, C-reactive protein, albumin, or leukocyte count with coronary heart disease: meta-analyses of prospective studies." *JAMA: The Journal of the American Medical Association* 279, no. 18 (May 13, 1998): 1477–1482.

Danesh, John, Sarah Lewington, Simon G. Thompson, Gordon D.O. Lowe, Rory Collins, J.B. Kostis, A.C. Wilson, et al. "Plasma fibrinogen level and the risk of major cardiovascular diseases and nonvascular mortality: an individual participant meta-analysis." *JAMA: The Journal of the American Medical Association* 294, no. 14 (October 12, 2005): 1799–1809.

Delavier, Frederic. *Strength Training Anatomy. 3rd ed.* Human Kinetics, 2010.

"Detection, evaluation and treatment of high blood cholesterol in adults ATP III final report." National Heart Lung and Blood Institute, n.d.

Di Angelantonio, Emanuele, Nadeem Sarwar, Philip Perry, Stephen Kaptoge, Kausik K Ray, Alexander Thompson, Angela M Wood, et al. "Major lipids, apolipoproteins, and risk of vascular disease." *JAMA: The Journal of the American Medical Association* 302, no. 18 (November 11, 2009): 1993–2000.

Erqou, Sebhat, Stephen Kaptoge, Philip L. Perry, Emanuele Di Angelantonio, Alexander Thompson, Ian R. White, Santica M. Marcovina, Rory Collins, Simon G. Thompson, and John Danesh. "Lipoprotein(a) concentration and the risk of coronary heart disease, stroke, and nonvascular mortality." *JAMA: The Journal of the American Medical Association* 302, no. 4 (July 22, 2009): 412–423.

"Exercise—Get weight loss advice, cardio and strength training workouts, information on how to get started and more," n.d. exercise.about.com/.

Farhadi, D. "Plasma homocysteine levels and mortality in patients with coronary artery disease." *The New England Journal of Medicine* 337, no. 22 (November 27, 1997): 1632; author reply 1632–1633.

Ferrannini, E., S.M. Haffner, B.D. Mitchell, and M.P. Stern. "Hyperinsulinaemia: the key feature of a cardiovascular and metabolic syndrome." *Diabetologia* 34, no. 6 (June 1991): 416–422.

"Fitness—MayoClinic.com," n.d. www.mayoclinic.com/health/fitness/MY00396.

Foster-Powell, Kaye, Susanna H.A. Holt, and Janette C. Brand-Miller. "International table of glycemic index and glycemic load values: 2002." *The American Journal of Clinical Nutrition* 76, no. 1 (July 1, 2002): 5–56.

Geberhiwot, Tarekegn, Angela Haddon, and Mourad Labib. "HbA1c predicts the likelihood of having impaired glucose tolerance in high-risk patients with normal fasting plasma glucose." *Annals of Clinical Biochemistry* 42, no. 3 (May

2005): 193–195.

Harris, T.B., L. Ferrucci, R.P. Tracy, M.C. Corti, S. Wacholder, W.H. Ettinger, H. Heimovitz, H.J. Cohen, and R. Wallace. "Associations of elevated interleukin-6 and C-reactive protein levels with mortality in the elderly." *The American Journal of Medicine* 106, no. 5 (May 1999): 506–512.

Kaptoge, S., I.R. White, S.G. Thompson, A.M. Wood, S. Lewington, G.D.O. Lowe, and J. Danesh. "Associations of plasma fibrinogen levels with established cardiovascular disease risk factors, inflammatory markers, and other characteristics: individual participant meta-analysis of 154,211 adults in 31 prospective studies: the fibrinogen studies collaboration." *American Journal of Epidemiology* 166, no. 8 (October 15, 2007): 867–879.

Koenig, W., M. Sund, M. Fröhlich, H.G. Fischer, H. Löwel, A. Döring, W.L. Hutchinson, and M.B. Pepys. "C—Reactive protein, a sensitive marker of inflammation, predicts future risk of coronary heart disease in initially healthy middle-aged men: results from the MONICA (Monitoring Trends and Determinants in Cardiovascular Disease) Augsburg Cohort Study, 1984 to 1992." *Circulation* 99, no. 2 (January 19, 1999): 237–242.

Lindeberg, S., M. Eliasson, B. Lindahl, and B. Ahrén. "Low serum insulin in traditional Pacific Islanders--the Kitava Study." *Metabolism: Clinical and Experimental* 48, no. 10 (October 1999): 1216–1219.

Nordestgaard, Børge G., M. John Chapman, Kausik Ray, Jan Borén, Felicita Andreotti, Gerald F. Watts, Henry Ginsberg, et al. "Lipoprotein(a) as a cardiovascular risk factor: current status." *European Heart Journal* (October 21, 2010). www.ncbi.nlm.nih.gov/pubmed/20965889.

"Physical activity and public health guidelines," n.d. www.acsm.org/AM/Template.cfm?Section=Home_Page&TEMPLATE=CM/HTMLDisplay.cfm&CONTENTID=7764.

Pradhan, A.D., J.E. Manson, N. Rifai, J.E. Buring, and P.M. Ridker.

"C-reactive protein, interleukin 6, and risk of developing type 2 diabetes mellitus." *JAMA: The Journal of the American Medical Association* 286, no. 3 (July 18, 2001): 327–334.

"Preventing and managing the global epidemic of obesity. Report of the World Health Organization consultation of obesity." World Health Organization, n.d.

Stampfer, M.J., M.R. Malinow, W.C. Willett, L.M. Newcomer, B. Upson, D. Ullmann, P.V. Tishler, and C.H. Hennekens. "A prospective study of plasma homocyst(e)ine and risk of myocardial infarction in US physicians." *JAMA: The Journal of the American Medical Association* 268, no. 7 (August 19, 1992): 877–881.

Stanger, O., W. Herrmann, K. Pietrzik, B. Fowler, J. Geisel, J. Dierkes, and M. Weger. "Clinical use and rational management of homocysteine, folic acid, and B vitamins in cardiovascular and thrombotic diseases." *Zeitschrift Für Kardiologie* 93, no. 6 (June 2004): 439–453.

"Stretching exercises.," n.d. physicaltherapy.about.com/od/flexibilityexercises/Stretching_Exercises.htm.

Tice, Jeffrey A., Warren Browner, Russell P. Tracy, and Steven R. Cummings. "The relation of C-reactive protein levels to total and cardiovascular mortality in older U.S. women." *The American Journal of Medicine* 114, no. 3 (February 15, 2003): 199–205.

Turner, R.C., R.R. Holman, D. Matthews, T.D. Hockaday, and J. Peto. "Insulin deficiency and insulin resistance interaction in diabetes: estimation of their relative contribution by feedback analysis from basal plasma insulin and glucose concentrations." *Metabolism: Clinical and Experimental* 28, no. 11 (November 1979): 1086–1096.

Wallace, Tara M., Jonathan C. Levy, and David R. Matthews. "Use and abuse of HOMA modeling." *Diabetes Care* 27, no. 6 (June 2004): 1487–1495.

"Weight training guidelines: ACSM recommendations and position stand," n.d. www.exrx.net/WeightTraining/Guidelines.html.

"WHO special issue—diet, nutrition and the prevention of chronic diseases: scientific background papers of the joint WHO/ FAO expert consultation, Geneva, 28 January–1 February 2002," n.d. www.who.int/nutrition/publications/obesity/ PHNvol7no1afeb2004/en/index.html.

Index

V

Vaillant, George 79
Vision 11, 13
Vitamin A 39, 44
Vitamin C 39, 71
Vitamin D 39–40, 67, 101
Vitamin E 39, 45

W

Weight Maintenance 32–34

Y

Yoga 82

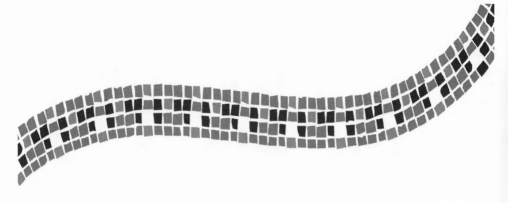

About the Author

Lorraine Maita, MD, is Board Certified in Internal Medicine and Anti-Aging and Regenerative Medicine and has over 18 years experience in Preventive Health and Wellness, Internal, Occupational and Travel Medicine and Executive Health. She served as Vice President and Chief Medical Officer at Prudential Financial, Medical Director on The Pfizer Health Leadership Team and Medical Director of North America for Johnson & Johnson Global Health Service and was an attending physician at St.Luke's/ Roosevelt Hospital, Emergency Department and Executive Health Examiners in New York City. She is a consultant for companies wanting to develop or enhance their employee and occupational health and wellness programs, and has a private practice in Short Hills, NJ.

Her programs have won recognition and awards such as The Pfizer Consumer Healthcare President's Innovation, The NJ Psychological Association Healthy Workplace, Outstanding Office Ergonomics from The Center for Office Technology, The NJ Heartsavers and The NJ Governors Safety Awards. She is author of "Vibrance for Life: How to Live Younger and Healthier" and a contributing author to Amazon's bestseller, "The Gratitude Book Project: 365 Days of Gratitude."

She is a Diplomate of the American College of Anti-Aging Medicine, and a member of the Age Management Medical Group, and the Executive Association of New Jersey. She has an appointment at Atlantic Health System's Morristown Memorial Hospital.

Made in the USA
Charleston, SC
07 August 2011